Wound Management

The *Essential Clinical Skills for Nurses* series focuses on key clinical skills for nurses and other health professionals. These concise, accessible books assume no prior knowledge and focus on core clinical skills, clearly presenting common clinical procedures and their rationale, together with the essential background theory. Their user-friendly format makes them an indispensable guide to clinical practice for all nurses, especially to student nurses and newly qualified staff.

Other titles in the *Essential Clinical Skills for Nurses* series:

Central Venous Access Devices
Lisa Dougherty
ISBN: 9781405119528

Clinical Assessment and Monitoring in Children
Diana Fergusson
ISBN: 9781405133388

Intravenous Therapy
Theresa Finlay
ISBN: 9780632064519

Respiratory Care
Caia Francis
ISBN: 9781405117173

Care of the Neurological Patient
Helen Iggulden
ISBN: 9781405117166

ECGs for Nurses
Phil Jevon
ISBN: 9780632058020

Monitoring the Critically Ill Patient
Second Edition
Phil Jevon and Beverley Ewens
ISBN: 9781405144407

Treating the Critically Ill Patient
Phil Jevon
ISBN: 9781405141727

Pain Management
Eileen Mann and Eloise Carr
ISBN: 9781405130714

Leg Ulcer Management
Christine Moffatt, Ruth Martin and Rachael Smithdale
ISBN: 9781405134767

Practical Resuscitation
Edited by Pam Moule and John Albarran
ISBN: 9781405116688

Pressure Area Care
Edited by Karen Ousey
ISBN: 9781405112253

Infection Prevention and Control
Christine Perry
ISBN: 9781405140386

Wound Management

Carol Dealey PhD MA BSc Hons RGN RCNT
Senior Research Fellow
University Hospital Birmingham NHS Foundation Trust
and University of Birmingham

and

Janice Cameron MPhil RGN ONC
Independent Nurse Advisor in Tissue Viability
(Formerly Clinical Nurse Specialist
in Wound Management)
Witney, Oxfordshire

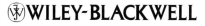WILEY-BLACKWELL

A John Wiley & Sons, Ltd., Publication

Blackwell Publishing was acquired by John Wiley & Sons in February 2007.
Blackwell's publishing programme has been merged with Wiley's global
Scientific, Technical, and Medical business to form Wiley-Blackwell.

Registered office
John Wiley & Sons Ltd, The Atrium, Southern Gate, Chichester, West Sussex,
PO19 8SQ, United Kingdom

Editorial office
9600 Garsington Road, Oxford, OX4 2DQ, United Kingdom
350 Main Street, Malden, MA 02148-5020, USA

For details of our global editorial offices, for customer services and
for information about how to apply for permission to reuse the
copyright material in this book please see our website at
www.wiley.com/wiley-blackwell.

Library of Congress Cataloging-in-Publication Data

Dealey, Carol.
Wound management / by Carol Dealey and Janice Cameron.
p. ; cm.
Includes bibliographical references and index.
ISBN-13: 978-1-4051-5541-0 (pbk. : alk. paper)
ISBN-10: 1-4051-5541-8 (pbk. : alk. paper) 1. Wounds and injuries –
Nursing.   2. Wound healing.   I. Cameron, Janice.   II. Title.
[DNLM: 1. Wounds and Injuries – nursing.   2. Wound
Healing.   3. Wounds and Injuries – therapy. WY 154 D2785w 2008]
RD93.95.D44 2008
617.1–dc22
2008002538

A catalogue record for this book is available from the British Library.

Set in 11/13 pt Palatino by SNP Best-set Typesetter Ltd., Hong Kong
Printed in Singapore by C.O.S. Printers Pte Ltd

i.e. 1 2008

Contents

Contributor

Deborah Hofman BA Hons Dip N RN
Clinical Nurse Specialist – Wound Management
Oxford Radcliffe Hospital NHS Trust
Churchill Hospital
Oxford

Introduction

ABOUT THIS BOOK

This book is primarily for pre-registration and newly qualified nurses. There is currently no recognised core curriculum for wound care in the pre-registration curriculum programme and wound management can often appear somewhat daunting to novice practitioners. The focus of this book is to educate practitioners in the general principles of wound care as well as techniques associated with the assessment, planning and management of different types of wound.

All aspects of healthcare delivery should be evidence based with a clear rationale for treatment. This book will provide the practitioner with an understanding of the principles of wound care and the ability to use a systematic approach to wound management.

LAYOUT OF THE BOOK

The book is set out in 10 chapters that follow a logical progression starting with the physiology of wound healing and continuing with information about the epidemiology of acute and chronic wounds. Using a holistic approach, the following seven chapters explore the principles and practice of assessing and managing a patient with a wound. The final chapter draws together the threads running throughout the book and shows how they can be applied in clinical practice.

A SYSTEMATIC APPROACH TO WOUND CARE

The information provided within this book will enable the practitioner to develop a systematic approach to learning in general and wound care in particular. The process can be divided into a series of steps thus enabling the practitioner to reach a logical conclusion regarding the most appropriate treatment plan. The steps are:

Step 1: assess the patient, wound and circumstances
Step 2: utilise existing information about the patient
Step 3: explore relevant current best practice
Step 4: make a clinical decision
Step 5: evaluate progress

EVIDENCE-BASED PRACTICE

Evidence-based practice means using current best evidence in a judicious manner to guide healthcare decisions with the aim of improving patient outcomes. In a number of instances the evidence has been used to develop clinical guidelines with recommendations for the assessment and management of specific wound types (see Table 1). The use of an evidence-based clinical guideline provides practitioners with recommendations for effective clinical practice, which can simplify their clinical decision-making, and practice that is not supported by good evidence is discouraged (McInnes *et al.*, 2000). There are national guidelines which many areas are adapting for local use (Graham *et al.*, 2005). The effectiveness of using clinical guidelines can be seen in terms of improved patient outcomes. For example, implementation of clinical guidelines for

Table 1 Different types of national and international clinical guidelines for wound care.

Wound type	Guideline issued by	Website address
Leg ulcers	Royal College of Nursing	www.rcn.org.uk
	Scottish Intercollegiate Guidelines Network (SIGN)	www.sign.ac.uk
Pressure ulcers	National Institute for Health and Clinical Excellence (NICE)	www.nice.org.uk
	European Pressure Ulcer Advisory Panel (EPUAP)	www.epuap.org
	National Pressure Ulcer Advisory Panel (NPUAP)	www.npuap.org
Diabetic foot ulcers	NICE	www.nice.org.uk
Surgical wound debridement	NICE	www.nice.org.uk

venous leg ulcers has been shown to improve healing rates and reduce costs (McGuckin *et al.*, 2002).

INTEGRATING THEORY AND PRACTICE

It is important to integrate theory and practice, and, therefore, there are case scenarios throughout the book for you to assess your knowledge. Using a systematic approach you can work through the different stages of assessment, planning and management using the knowledge you have gained from the preceding chapter. The suggested management section after each case scenario discusses the various options, where you can compare your answers. All qualified nurses are accountable for their actions and as such should ensure that they have the required knowledge to provide optimum care for their patients.

REFERENCES

Graham, I.D., Harrison, M.B., Lorimer, K., Piercianowski, T., Friedberg, E., Buchanan, M. & Harris, C. (2005) Adapting national and international leg ulcer practice guidelines for local use. *Advances in Skin and Wound Care* **18**(6): 307–318.

McGuckin, M., Waterman, R., Brooks, J., Cherry, G., Porten, L., Hurley, S. & Kerstein, M.D. (2002) Validation of venous leg ulcer guidelines in the United States and United Kingdom. *American Journal of Surgery* **183**(2): 132–137.

McInnes, E., Cullum, N., Nelson, E.A., Luker, K. & Duff, L.A. (2000) The development of a national guideline on the management of leg ulcers. *Journal of Clinical Nursing* **9**(2): 208–217.

Wound Physiology

INTRODUCTION

A wound is a loss of continuity of the skin, which may occur as a result of injury, impaired blood supply or deliberate wounding such as surgery. Healing time varies according to the type of injury and the extent of tissue loss. Superficial wounds in which only epithelial tissue is damaged require a relatively short time to heal, whereas healing takes longer and is more complex in deep wounds in which vessels have been damaged.

It is essential that those involved in the care and management of wounds should have at the very least a basic understanding of the physiology of the natural processes involved in wound healing. Understanding and recognition of the different stages of healing will assist the healthcare practitioner in assessment and decision-making in the care and management of the patient with a wound. This chapter presents an overview of the physiology of wound healing. The structure and functions of the skin are described in Chapter 6.

HEALING BY PRIMARY AND SECONDARY INTENTION

- Healing by primary intention is when there is no tissue loss and the skin edges are brought together, such as in a sutured wound.

- Healing by secondary intention is when there is tissue loss and the skin edges are far apart. The wound heals from the base upwards. Examples of this type of wound are a pressure ulcer, a leg ulcer or an open excision such as an abdominal wound.

PARTIAL AND FULL THICKNESS WOUNDS

- Superficial wounds involving the epidermis (and sometimes the upper dermis), leaving lower levels of skin intact, are referred to as partial thickness wounds (Fig. 1.1). Examples are a simple skin abrasion or a donor site from a split thickness skin graft. Epithelial cells migrate towards each other from the

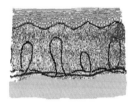

Normal skin

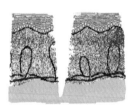

Incision wound

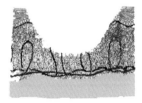

Partial thickness wound

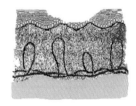

Superficial wound

Fig. 1.1 Types of wound. Reproduced with kind permission from Dr George Cherry.

edges of the wound and from the hair follicles, seba-ceous glands and sweat glands. This part of the healing process is known as epithelialisation.
• In a full thickness wound all of the dermis is destroyed and the deeper layers may also be involved. These wounds heal by secondary inten-tion, in which granulation tissue is formed to fill the wound space and new epidermis grows over it (Knighton *et al.*, 1990).

THE HEALING PROCESS
The healing process occurs as a natural response to injury and initiates a highly complex cascade of events, which in the normal healing wound occur in an orderly and timely fashion, resulting in skin repair. Wound healing consists of four main phases that overlap each other and are intricately linked:

• Inflammation
• Reconstruction (granulation tissue production)
• Re-epithelialisation
• Maturation

Phase I – inflammation
Immediately following injury, the body's defence mechanisms produce an inflammatory response. This initial phase of healing lasts up to 4–6 days post wounding. Injured blood vessels bleed into the wound and platelets adhere to exposed collagen in the sub-endothelial layers of the walls of the damaged blood vessels. The platelets flatten and release substances, including proteins, which cause the platelets to become sticky. Fibrin combines with the platelets and trapped

erythrocytes to form a clot, thus occluding the damaged blood vessels (Cooper, 1990).

Activated platelets release growth factors, including platelet-derived growth factor (PDGF) and epidermal growth factor (EGF). The term 'growth factors' is used to describe the various proteins involved in co-ordinating the cascade of events involved in wound healing (Graham, 1998). However, the number of growth factors that relate to wound healing is unclear and there is ongoing research in this field. Growth factors have a major role in providing the means of cell communication throughout the wound healing process. PDGF supports the initial inflammatory stages of healing and also has an important role in the formation of granulation tissue, collagen and ground substance. EGF has a significant role in epithelialisation and in the formation of granulation tissue (Kunimoto, 2001). These growth factors act as chemoattractant chemicals, which facilitate the migration of neutrophils to the area. Neutrophils and monocytes can be found in the wound on the first day and are responsible for initiating the wound cleansing process by removing bacteria, devitalised tissue and debris from the wound using a process known as phagocytosis (Ovington & Schultz, 2004).

Inflammation leads to an increase in vasodilation and vessel permeability. Histamine and serotonin are released, which increase capillary permeability, allowing plasma leakage, which in turn leads to accumulation of fluid in adjacent tissues (Thomas, 1997). The increased blood supply and oedema produce the inflammatory appearance of erythema and swelling, together with heat, and the patient experiences localised pain. Excessive fluid drains from the wound tissue as exudate. Wound fluid from acute wounds is rich in growth factors that have been shown to promote tissue repair (Chen *et al.*, 1992).

At the end of the acute inflammatory phase neutrophils decay and are themselves phagocytosed by macrophages that have matured from monocytes. Macrophages continue to phagocytose and digest bacteria, wound debris and necrotic tissue performing autolytic debridement of the wound (Moore, 2003).

Phase II – reconstruction (granulation tissue production)

Macrophages secrete growth factors crucial to wound healing and facilitate angiogenesis (the growth of new blood vessels from damaged vessels), cell migration and proliferation, the restoration of the nutrient blood supply and synthesis of new tissue (Cooper, 1990; Brem, 2001). Oxygen is vital to this process and macrophages can be inactivated by oxygen pressure below 30 mm Hg (Cherry *et al.*, 2000). Fibroblast growth factor (FGF) is released by macrophages and fibroblasts and is an important growth factor for angiogenesis and the formation of new granulation tissue (Kunimoto, 2001). The acute wound fluid stimulates fibroblast and endothelial cell growth (Katz *et al.*, 1991). Fibroblasts have a key role in this phase of healing (Harding *et al.*, 2002). They synthesise and secrete the collagen and ground substance, forming a provisional wound bed matrix (the extracellular matrix), which acts as the scaffolding for repair (Greener *et al.*, 2005).

The wound surface has a relatively low oxygen tension, encouraging the process of angiogenesis, where new capillaries sprout from blood vessels at the wound periphery (Silver, 1985). They then join together to form a network of capillary loops, infiltrating the extracellular matrix, and supplying oxygen and essential nutrients to the wound (Cutting & Tong, 2003).

The new tissue, composed of the capillary loops, the supporting collagen and the ground substance, is red in colour and has a slightly rough, granular appearance. This is what is termed 'granulation tissue'. In wounds healing by secondary intention granulation tissue can be seen as it gradually fills the wound cavity. As the wound fills with new tissue and a capillary network is formed, the numbers of macrophages and fibroblasts gradually reduce (Dealey, 2005).

Healing may be delayed if infection is present. Healing may also be compromised if damage has been caused due to an unsuitable dressing being applied to the wound.

Wound contraction
Contraction is a normal part of wound healing that may start at around the fifth or sixth day. In this process, cellular forces pull the wound edges towards the centre of the wound. Fibroblasts have been found to be particularly important in wound contraction (Viennet *et al.*, 2004). Contraction can reduce the surface area of open wounds by as much as 40–80% of the closure (Irvin, 1987).

Phase III – re-epithelialisation
Macrophages release EGF, which stimulates both the proliferation and migration of epithelial cells.

Keratinocytes migrate from the wound edges to cover the surface and re-form the layers of destroyed epithelium. Keratinocytes are also largely responsible for reconstituting the basement membrane of the dermal–epidermal junction (Hughes, 2002).

The epithelial cells migrate and proliferate from the wound edges and cover viable tissue with a leap-frogging action. The cells multiply and divide by mitosis and migrate across the surface until they meet in the middle of the wound (Dealey, 2005).

Phase IV – maturation

During the maturation phase the components of the extracellular matrix change and collagen fibres are restructured, becoming thicker and stronger, giving greater tensile strength to the new tissues over time (Hughes, 2002). A newly healed surgical wound has little tensile strength, but will gradually increase to about 50% of the normal tissue after 3 months (Forester *et al.*, 1970). Collagen is constantly degraded and new collagen synthesised. Remodelling of the collagen fibres is a lengthy process that continues for months or years after healing, allowing the wound to continue to strengthen (Moore, 2003). Scars usually flatten and soften and eventually fade (Hughes, 2002). Abnormal scarring may occur if collagen production occurs at a greater rate than its destruction (Smith, 2005).

ACUTE AND CHRONIC WOUNDS

An acute wound is one that heals within a relatively short time frame without complications. The healing process is automatically triggered into action and destroyed tissue is replace by living tissue. A wound becomes chronic when there is failure of the normal processes of healing, as a result of various underlying problems and pathological conditions. A chronic wound is slow to heal taking months or even years. Falanga (2002) describes chronic wounds as having a complex life of their own.

Wound exudate

Studies on wound exudate have established differences between acute wound fluid and chronic wound fluid. The production of wound exudate is a normal part of the inflammatory process (Thomas, 1997). Wound fluid from acute wounds has beneficial properties that have been shown to stimulate cell proliferation and thus plays an essential part in the healing process (Katz *et al.*, 1991; Chen *et al.*, 1992). Chronic wounds have a prolonged inflammatory response leading to increased and prolonged production of wound exudate that interferes with healing (Moore, 1999; Hart, 2002). Wound fluid from chronic wounds has been shown to have a damaging effect on healing due to sustained high levels of tissue-destructive enzymes (Trengove *et al.*, 1999; Krishnamoorthy *et al.*, 2001). In a normal healing acute wound, high levels of protease activity, which is responsible for clearing the debris from the wound, decrease as the wound heals, whereas in chronic wound fluid protease activity remains increased (Wysocki *et al.*, 1993; Yager & Nwomeh, 1999). Research suggests that wound exudate in non-healing chronic wounds has a damaging effect on wound healing because of the impaired proliferation of key cells in the healing process (Hoffman *et al.*, 1998; Trengove *et al.*, 1999; Krishnamoorthy *et al.*, 2001;

Table 1.1 Differences between acute and chronic wounds.

Acute wounds	Chronic wounds
Heal within a relatively short time frame	Slow to heal
Heal without complications	Complications due to various underlying problems and pathological conditions
Normal inflammatory response	Prolonged inflammatory response
Exudate production decreases as wound heals	Increased and prolonged production of wound exudate
Acute wound fluid (AWF) stimulates cell proliferation	Chronic wound fluid (CWF) has sustained high levels of tissue destructive enzymes
Decrease in protease activity in AWF as wound heals	Increased protease activity in CWF contributes to degradation of cell adhesion proteins required for tissue repair

Drinkwater *et al.*, 2002). Table 1.1 summarises how the healing process is affected in acute and chronic wounds.

Key points

- Wound healing consists of four main phases that overlap each other and are intricately linked.
- The initial inflammatory response is followed by tissue proliferation.

Continued

- The process of autolysis occurs in the wound (natural degradation of devitalised tissue).
- Granulation tissue production leads to formation of new blood vessels (angiogenesis).
- Contraction is a normal part of wound healing that reduces the surface area of open wounds.
- Re-epithelialisation resurfaces the wound. Epithelial cells migrate towards each other from the edges of the wound, hair follicles, sebaceous glands and sweat glands.
- In the maturation phase components of the extracellular matrix change and collagen fibres are restructured, becoming thicker and stronger, and gradually giving greater tensile strength to the new tissues.
- Acute wounds heal within a relatively short time frame without complications.
- Chronic wounds are slow to heal, taking months or years.
- Experimental studies have identified differences in acute and chronic wound fluid. Acute wound fluid is essential in promoting tissue repair whereas chronic wound fluid has a potential damaging effect.

SUMMARY

This chapter has focused on giving you a basic understanding of the healing process and the differences between an acute wound and a chronic wound. You should now use the knowledge you have gained from reading this chapter to undertake the following exercise.

Exercise 1.1

Case scenario

You have been given the following assignment, which requires you to explain to a patient how a wound heals following surgery. Mr Roy Jones, 72 years, was a teacher at the local secondary school where he taught physics and has been retired for 10 years. Mr Jones has been admitted for a hip replacement. Prior to problems with his hip he was a keen walker. He is an articulate, thoughtful man who likes to read and do puzzles to keep his mind active. Mr Jones has been reading an article in a magazine about wounds and has become very interested in the physiology of the healing process. Your assignment requires you to explain to him how his wound is going to heal.

Using a systematic approach, think about how you will go about this and what level of detail you should give to the patient.

Step 1: assess the patient, wound and circumstances
Mr Jones is about to have surgery for a hip replacement. Consider what you have learned in this chapter and identify the specific aspects of healing in a surgical wound. Consider how much detailed information you would give to this patient.

Step 2: utilise existing information about the patient
Consider the level of knowledge Mr Jones already has.

Step 3: explore relevant current best practice
Identify where there is evidence available to support what you will say.

Continued

Step 4: make a clinical decision
You should now tailor the information you have gained to meet the specific needs of this patient.

Step 5: evaluate progress
Think about how you would be able to determine if the information you have given has met the patient's requirements.

Suggested management

In Exercise 1.1, Mr Jones has a very active mind and is seeking further information. This patient is a retired teacher of physics and would easily understand a basic description of the physiology of the healing process. Patient information leaflets are a valuable resource for giving explanations to patients, but they would probably not go into enough detail for this patient. You have been told that Mr Jones has already gained some information from the article about wounds that he was reading and this would be your starting point. You could explain that a surgical wound heals by primary intention and what this means. You could then go on to describe the healing process using the key points given in this chapter as your base and expand this as required. You should always use up-to-date evidence-based material when undertaking your assignments and also in practice. Such information can be gained from relevant textbooks and journals.

After explaining something to a patient you should always ask them if they have understood what you have told them, whether they would like to ask any questions and if they require further information. You would probably find that someone like the patient described here would ask questions if he wanted further information. He may wish to borrow a library book for further reading around the subject and you could suggest a suitable one.

REFERENCES

Brem, H. (2001) Specific paradigm for wound bed preparation in chronic wounds. In: Cherry, G.W., Harding, K.G. & Ryan, T.J. (eds) *Wound Bed Preparation.* International Congress and Symposium Series No. 250. London, Royal Society of Medicine Press.

Chen, W.Y.J., Rogers, A.A. & Lydon, M.J. (1992) Characterization of biologic properties of wound fluid collected during early stages of wound healing. *Journal of Investigative Dermatology* **99**: 559–564.

Cherry, G.W., Hughes, M.A., Ferguson, M.W.J. & Leaper, D.J. (2000) Wound healing. In: Morris, P.J. & Wood, W.C. (eds) *Oxford Textbook of Surgery, Second Edition.* Oxford, Oxford University Press.

Cooper, D.M. (1990) The physiology of wound healing: an overview. In: Krasner, D. (ed.) *Chronic Wound Care: A Clinical Source Book for Healthcare Professionals.* Pennsylvania, Health Management Publications.

Cutting, K. & Tong, A. (2003) Wound physiology and moist wound healing. *Clinical Education in Wound Management Series.* Holsworthy, Medical Communications.

Dealey, C. (2005) *The Care of Wounds: A Guide for Nurses, Third Edition.* Oxford, Blackwell Science.

Drinkwater, S.L., Smith, A., Sawyer, B.M. & Barnard, K.G. (2002) Effect of venous ulcer exudates on angiogenesis in vitro. *British Journal of Surgery* **89**(6): 709–713.

Falanga, V. (2002) The clinical relevance of wound bed preparation. In: Falanga, V. & Harding, K. (eds) *The Clinical Relevance of Wound Bed Preparation.* Berlin, Springer-Verlag.

Forester, J.C., Zederfeldt, B.H., Hayes, T.L. & Hunt, T.K. (1970) Tape-closed and sutured wounds: a comparison by tensiometry and scanning electron microscopy. *British Journal of Surgery* **57**: 729–737.

Graham A. (1998) The use of growth factors in clinical practice. *Journal of Wound Care* **7**(9): 464–466.

Greener, B., Hughes, A.A., Bannister, N.P. & Douglass, J. (2005) Proteases and pH in chronic wounds. *Journal of Wound Care* **14**(2): 59–61.

Harding, K.G., Morris, H.L. & Patel, G.K. (2002) Healing chronic wounds. *British Medical Journal* **324**: 160–163.

Hart, J. (2002) Inflammation 1: its role in acute wounds. *Journal of Wound Care* **11**(6): 205–209.

Hoffman, R., Starkey, S. & Coad, J. (1998) Wound fluid from venous leg ulcers degrades plasminogen and reduces plasmin generation by keratinocytes. *Journal of Investigative Dermatology* **111**: 1140–1144.

Hughes, M. (2002) The science of wound healing. *The Oxford European Wound Healing Course Hand Book.* Positif Press, Oxford.

Irvin, T.T. (1987) The principles of wound healing. *Surgery* **1**: 1112–1115.

Katz, M.H., Alvarz, A.F., Kirsner, R.S., Eaglestein, W.H. & Falanga, V. (1991) Human wound fluid from acute wounds stimulates fibroblast and endothelial cell growth. *Journal of the American Academy of Dermatology* **25**(6 part 1): 1054–1058.

Knighton, D.R., Fiegel, V.D. & Doucette, M.M. (1990) Wound repair: the growth factor revolution. In: Krasner, D. (ed.) *Chronic Wound Care. A Clinical Source Book for Healthcare Professionals.* Pennsylvania, Health Management Publications.

Krishnamoorthy, L., Morris, H.L. & Harding, K.G. (2001) A dynamic regulator: the role of growth factors in tissue repair. *Journal of Wound Care* **10**(4): 99–101.

Kunimoto, B.T. (2001) Growth factors in wound healing. In: Krasner, D.L., Rodeheaver, G.T. & Sibald, R.G. (eds)

Chronic Wound Care. A Clinical Source Book for Healthcare Professionals, Third Edition. Wayne, PA, HMP Communications.

Moore, K. (1999) Cell biology of chronic wounds: the role of inflammation. *Journal of Wound Care* **8**(7): 345–348.

Moore, K. (2003) Wound physiology: from healing to chronicity. *Journal of Wound Care* **12**(10) Johnson & Johnson supplement: part 2.

Ovington, L.G. & Schultz, G.S. (2004) The physiology of wound healing. In: Morison, M.J., Ovington, L.G. & Wilkie, K. (eds) *Chronic Wound Care: A Problem Based Learning Approach.* Edinburgh, Mosby.

Silver, I.A. (1985) Oxygen and tissue repair. In: Ryan, T.J. (ed). *An Environment for Healing: The Role of Occlusion.* International Congress and Symposium Series No. 88. London, Royal Society of Medicine.

Smith, F.R. (2005) Causes and treatment options for abnormal scar tissue. *Journal of Wound Care* **14**(2): 49–52.

Thomas, S. (1997) Assessment and management of wound exudate. *Journal of Wound Care* **6**(7): 327–330.

Trengove, N.J., Stacey, M.C., MacAuley, S., Bennett, N., Gibson, J., Burslem, F., Murphy, G. & Schultz, G. (1999) Analysis of the acute and chronic wound environments: the role of proteases and their inhibitors. *Wound Repair Regeneration* **7**: 42–52.

Viennet, C., Gabiot, A.C., Gharbi, T., Bride, J. & Humbert, P. (2004) Comparing the contractual properties of human fibroblasts in leg ulcers with normal fibroblasts. *Journal of Wound Care* **13**(9): 358–361.

Wysocki, A.B., Staiano-Coico, L. & Grinnell, F. (1993) Wound fluid from chronic leg ulcers contains elevated levels of metalloproteinases, MMP-2 and MMP-9. *Journal of Investigative Dermatology* **101**: 64–68.

Yager, D.R. & Nwomeh, B.C. (1999) The proteolytic environment of chronic wounds. *Wound Repair and Regeneration* **7**(6): 433–441.

The Epidemiology of Acute and Chronic Wounds

INTRODUCTION

Nurses may come in contact with a variety of wounds. They are generally categorised as acute or chronic wounds. Acute wounds generally heal promptly whereas chronic wounds do not heal easily and are often subject to complications. This chapter will consider the epidemiology of both acute and chronic wounds. Epidemiology is the study of the incidence and distribution of diseases in human populations, in other words:

- What types are there? (Types of wounds)
- How many are there? (Prevalence and incidence)
- Where are they and who looks after them? (Hospital or community)

TYPES OF WOUNDS AND THEIR INCIDENCE AND PREVALENCE

The different types of wounds are summarised in Table 2.1 and described in more detail here. In order to understand the significance of the different wound types it is useful to be aware of their numbers. In healthcare this is measured in terms of prevalence and incidence. Prevalence means the total number of cases with a specific condition within a given population at a particular point in time. Incidence means the number

Table 2.1 Different wound types.

Category	Type
Acute	Surgical wounds
	Traumatic wounds
	Burn injury
Chronic	Pressure ulcer
	Leg ulcer
	Diabetic foot ulcer
	Malignant fungating wounds

of new cases with a specific condition occurring within a given population, usually measured over a period of time. An example of a prevalence survey is the number of patients with pressure ulcers in a hospital on a particular day; this would include patients who were admitted with pressure ulcers as well as those who developed them while in the hospital. The prevalence rate is calculated as a percentage of the number of inpatients on the day of the survey. On the other hand, measurement of incidence would only include those patients who develop pressure ulcers while in hospital and is usually measured over a period of time. Incidence is calculated as a percentage of the number of admissions over the period of time being measured.

ACUTE WOUNDS
Surgical wounds

Surgical wounds are, fairly obviously, as a result of a surgical procedure. They can vary greatly in size and can occur on any part of the body. Most surgical wounds have the skin edges held together by sutures, clips or tape. A smaller number may be left open to heal from the bottom up or for suturing a few days later. These wounds are usually associated with infection, for example an abscess. The numbers of operations being undertaken are counted in relation to government targets and for planning future care delivery, but it is not considered necessary to count the number of surgical wounds for epidemiological studies, as they are intentional wounds undertaken to repair a problem. However, the incidence of surgical wound infection is monitored as this is a complication that can have serious implications for the patient as well as costing a great deal to treat.

When monitoring the rate of infection in surgical wounds it is usual to divide wounds into different categories according to the potential for developing wound infection. Table 2.2 shows the different categories and the infection rates found in a large study undertaken over 10 years (Cruse & Foord, 1980). It demonstrates how the potential for infection varies and why prophylactic antibiotics may be given routinely to prevent infection in high-risk operations such as following traumatic injury. This study was the first large survey of its kind and has set the standard for others that have followed. A review of prevalence and incidence studies across Europe by Leaper *et al.* (2004) found considerable variation in rates, partially due to different methods of data collection. Figures ranged from 1.5% to 20% and the associated costs were estimated to be between 1.47 and 19.1 billion euros. However, Alfonso *et al.* (2007) suggest that this is likely

Table 2.2 Classification of surgical wounds to measure infection rates.

Category	Description	Infection rate (%)
Clean	Surgery where there is no sign of infection or inflammation, there is no break in asepsis, and hollow organs such as the bowel are not entered	1.5
Clean-contaminated	Surgery where a hollow organ is entered, but there has been only minimal spillage of the contents	7.7
Contaminated	Surgery where a hollow organ is opened with gross spillage, where there is acute inflammation without pus (e.g. inflamed appendix), where there is a major break in asepsis or in traumatic wounds less than 4 hours old	15.2
Dirty	Surgery where pus or perforation is found (e.g. perforated appendix) or traumatic injury more than 4 hours old	40

Based on Cruse & Foord (1980).

to be an underestimate as the true cost of surgical wound infection should also include the impact on society of temporary incapacity of the individual and even an estimation of years of productive life lost for those who die as a result of their infection. They calculated that the health costs amounted to only 10% of the total figure (US$97 433) and the remainder were socio-labour costs.

Traumatic injuries

Traumatic wounds are caused by accidental or malicious injury. Major traumatic wounds require surgery and so become translated into surgical wounds. Minor traumatic injury includes cuts, abrasions, lacerations, skin tears, animal or human bites and finger-tip injuries. The more serious of these injuries require treatment in an accident and emergency department (A&E). In 2003 there were 12.7 million visits to A&Es in England alone and around a fifth were sufficiently serious as to require hospital admission (National Audit Office, 2004).

Abrasions can be described as a superficial injury where the skin surface is rubbed or torn (Dealey, 2005). This type of injury most commonly occurs from falling onto a rough or gravelled surface.

Lacerations are penetrating wounds with a jagged edge. They are caused by sharp objects such as glass or knives or damage from a blunt instrument that causes tearing of the skin and possibly the tissues below. The commonest position for a laceration is just below the knee and this is called a pre-tibial laceration. Davis *et al.* (2004) found that for every 1000 attendances at A&Es in one region, 5.2 attendances were for treatments of pre-tibial lacerations.

Skin tears look similar to lacerations but are caused by friction and/or shearing forces and occur in people with thin fragile skin, particularly the elderly. They mostly occur on the arms or legs and may be caused by rough handling. Little is known about the incidence of skin tears in the UK, but it has been suggested that in the USA in one year as many as 1.5 million nursing home residents will have a skin tear (Thomas *et al.*, 1999).

Animal and human bites cause bruises, cuts, lacerations or puncture wounds and represent 1% of visits to A&Es each year (Medeiros & Saconato, 2004). Although most of the publicity around these bites concerns dog bites, patients have also been bitten by cats, rats, squirrels and snakes. Human bites predominantly occur from fighting and may be found on the hand as a result of a punch to the mouth as well as on the torso.

Finger-tip injuries most commonly occur in young children who get their fingers crushed in doors. The incidence for this type of injury may be as high as 14% in those under 13 years of age (Buckles, 1985).

Burn injury
Burn wounds are also traumatic injuries, but as they need specialised care they are managed differently from other types of trauma wounds (Dealey, 2005). There are four causes of burns:

- Thermal – fire or hot fluids
- Electrical
- Chemical – spillage of corrosive substances
- Radiation – skin reaction to radiotherapy treatment

Severe burn injuries are potentially fatal. A national review of burn care provision in the UK (National

Burn Care Review Committee, 2001) reported that about 300 in 250 000 sufferers die each year from their injuries. Although small burns may be treated simply by first aid in the home or at work, about 175 000 people attend A&E each year and of these, 13 000 will require admission to hospital. Sadly, some burn injuries are caused by non-accidental injury which may be self-inflicted or inflicted by others. Approximately 10% of the burns suffered by children are caused by physical abuse (Gordon & Goodwin, 1997).

CHRONIC WOUNDS
Pressure ulcers

Pressure ulcers have been defined as: 'an area of localised damage to the skin and underlying tissues caused by pressure, shear, friction or a combination of these' (European Pressure Ulcer Advisory Panel, 1999). They are also known as pressure ulcers, bed sores or decubitus ulcers. The cause of pressure ulcers is multifactorial as the external factors of pressure, friction and shear combine with factors within the patient to precipitate the damage. These intrinsic factors include age, immobility, loss of sensation, incontinence and poor nutrition. There are numerous problems in comparing the prevalence and incidence of pressure ulcers as many different methods have been used (Lahmann et al., 2006). A large study of 5947 patients across five European countries found a prevalence rate of 18.1% (Clark et al., 2003). However, as the study itself was actually a pilot study, this does not represent an indication of actual prevalence in Europe, but it does show it is a considerable problem.

Leg ulcers

Leg ulcers are wounds on the leg or foot that fail to heal within 6 weeks (Dale *et al.*, 1983). There are several different causes of leg ulcers but the most common is damage to either the veins or the arteries of the leg. Many people who have leg ulcers find that not only do they take a long time to heal but they are also liable to re-occur. In the Western world, recurrent leg ulceration occurs in 1–2% of the adult population (Briggs & Closs, 2003). A survey by Moffatt *et al.* (2004) found that 55% of those with leg ulcers had had them for more than 12 months.

Diabetic foot ulcers

People with diabetes are vulnerable to the development of ulcers on their feet. These ulcers can occur as a result of damage to the local nervous system causing loss of sensation, known as peripheral neuropathy, or constriction of the small arteries in the foot, or a combination of the two. Jeffcoate and Harding (2003) stated that people with diabetes have a lifetime risk of about 15% of developing an ulcer. The major complication of diabetic foot ulceration is that of amputation. This can be amputation of a toe or part of the foot or major amputation of the affected limb. Jeffcoate and Harding (2003) quote an incidence rate of 0.5–5.0/1000 patients with diabetes for major amputations and an associated perioperative mortality rate of 9–15% in this group.

Malignant fungating wounds

Malignant fungating wounds occur when a cancerous growth erupts through the skin to the body surface causing an ulcerous surface. They are mostly associated with cancers that are near the body surface such as cancers of the breast, skin, vulva, head and neck or the bladder. They can also be found in cancers that have spread from the original site, known as metastatic cancer. Very little is known of the incidence of these wounds, but Haisfield-Wolfe and Rund (1997) estimate that 5–10% of patients with metastatic cancer will develop a fungating wound.

WHERE CAN PATIENTS WITH WOUNDS BE FOUND?

A wide range of healthcare professionals are involved in some aspect of the provision of wound care as patients with wounds can be found in hospital or in the community. There are also nurses who specialise in wound care, usually called 'tissue viability nurse specialists', and they may cover both hospital and community so may see patients in hospital, in a clinic or in their own home. Table 2.3 provides a list of different healthcare professionals and the role they may play in wound care. Whoever is involved, it is important to work as a team to ensure effective provision of care.

Theoretically, it can be suggested that some wounds will only be found in hospital or in the community, but this is rarely the case. For example, a patient with minor traumatic injuries may attend A&E in the first instance, but then be referred back to their GP for removal of sutures. Alternatively, patients with leg ulcers are predominantly cared for by community nurses, but may be referred to a vascular surgeon or a dermatologist in the local hospital for advice if the ulcer is not healing.

Table 2.3 Healthcare professionals providing wound care.

Profession	Specialty	Comment
Nurses	A&E	Traumatic wounds
	Hospital nurses	Wide variety of wounds, but may have specialist knowledge of one particular type of wound
	Community and practice nurses	Wide variety of wounds, often have specialist knowledge of leg ulcer care
	Tissue viability nurse specialists	Specialise in wound care and provide service across hospital and/or community. May run an equipment store with pressure relieving mattresses etc.
Doctors	GPs	May need to provide support to the community nurse if wound develops complications
	A&E surgeons	Provide first-line treatment for trauma wounds
	Hospital physicians (especially dermatologists, diabetologists and geriatricians)	Chronic wounds
	Hospital surgeons	Wide variety of wounds found in all specialties

Continued

Table 2.3 *Continued*

Profession	Specialty	Comment
Pharmacists		Provision of wound care products in either hospital or community
Podiatrists (chiropodists)		Provide foot care including foot ulcers of all types
Orthotists		Provides specialised footwear and appliances
Dieticians		Dietary advice for those with specific conditions, e.g. diabetes. Also give advice to patients with large wounds

The wide distribution of patients with wounds indicates that all nurses need to have general skill in wound care as well as specialist knowledge relevant to their own sphere of practice.

Key points

- Epidemiological studies of wounds measure them using the terms prevalence and incidence.
- *Prevalence*: the total number of cases with a specific condition within a given population at a particular point in time.

Continued

- *Incidence*: the number of new cases with a specific condition occurring within a given population, usually measured over a period of time.
- Wounds are categorised as acute wounds, such as surgical and traumatic wounds, and chronic wounds, such as pressure and leg ulcers.
- Patients with wounds are cared for in many different circumstances – in a hospital ward, outpatient department, at home or in general practice.

SUMMARY

This chapter has provided an overview of the epidemiology of all types of wounds, where they may be found and the healthcare personnel involved in the care of wounds. You should now use the knowledge you have gained from reading this chapter to undertake the following exercise.

Exercise 2.1

Case scenario

Len Jones is a fit, active 53-year-old man, who works as a labourer on a building site. He has to wear industrial boots for work. One day, after removing his boots he notices that he has a small wound on the sole of his foot and goes to see his general practitioner (GP). Whom might the GP ask to assist in providing wound care for this patient?

Continued

27

> ***Using a systematic approach think about how you will determine who will be involved in this patient's care.***
>
> *Step 1: assess the patient, wound and circumstances*
> Len has an ulcer on the sole of his foot and has to wear industrial boots at work over the area of the wound.
>
> *Step 2: utilise existing information about the patient*
> You know Len's age and that he is fit and active and the type of job that he does.
>
> *Step 3: explore relevant current best practice*
> Len is able to attend his local health centre for treatment. Consider who the most appropriate person would be to undertake the dressing.
>
> *Step 4: make a clinical decision*
> You need to consider that Len has to wear industrial boots at work. Will they still fit when the dressing is in place? Who could give additional advice about this?
>
> *Step 5: evaluate progress*
> Who will evaluate whether Len's wound is healing?

Suggested management

Len is a fit and active man and therefore can easily attend the local health centre. The most appropriate person for him to see is the practice nurse, as she will have experience in dressing wounds. The bulk of the dressing may affect the fit of Len's footwear, which could cause his boot to rub elsewhere on his foot. The most appropriate person who has expertise in addressing problems with footwear is the podiatrist. If different footwear is required the orthotist may also be involved. The practice nurse will continue to do Len's dressing and therefore will be the person to monitor and evaluate his progress.

REFERENCES

Alfonso, J.L., Pereperez, S.B., Canovez, J.M., Martinez, M.M. & Martin-Moreno, J.M. (2007) Are we really seeing the total costs of surgical site infection? A Spanish study. *Wound Repair and Regeneration* **15**(4): 474–481.

Briggs, M. & Closs, S.J. (2003) The prevalence of leg ulceration: a review of the literature. *EWMA Journal* **3**(2): 14–20.

Buckles, E. (1985) Wound care in accident and emergency. *Nursing* **2**(suppl)(42): 3–5.

Clark, M., Bours, G. & Defloor, T. (2003) The prevalence of pressure ulcers in Europe. *Hospital Decisions*, **Winter** 2003/2004.

Cruse, P.J.E. & Foord, R. (1980) The epidemiology of wound infection, a ten-year prospective study of 62,939 wounds. *Surgical Clinics of North America* **60**(1): 27–40.

Dale, J.J., Callum, M.J., Ruckley, C., Harper, D.R. & Berrey, P.N. (1983) Chronic ulcers of the leg: a study of prevalence in a Scottish community. *Edinburgh Health Bulletin* **41**: 310–314.

Davis, A., Chester, D., Allison, K. & Davison, P. (2004) A survey of how a region's A&E units manage pretibial lacerations. *Journal of Wound Care* **13**(1): 5–7.

Dealey, C. (2005) *The Care of Wounds, Third Edition.* Oxford, Blackwell Science.

European Pressure Ulcer Advisory Panel (1999) Pressure ulcer treatment guidelines. *EPUAP Review* **1**(2): 31–33.

Gordon, M. & Goodwin, C.W. (1997) Initial assessment, management and stabilisation. *Nursing Clinics of North America* **32**(2): 237–249.

Haisfield-Wolfe, M.A. & Rund, C. (1997) Malignant cutaneous wounds: a management protocol. *Ostomy and Wound Management* **43**: 56–66.

Jeffcoate, W.J. & Harding, K.G. (2003) Diabetic foot ulcers. *The Lancet* **361**(9368): 1545–1551.

Lahmann, N., Halfens, R.J. & Dassen, T. (2006) Effect of non-response bias in pressure ulcer prevalence studies. *Journal of Advanced Nursing* **55**(2): 230–236.

Leaper, D.J., Van Goor, H., Reilly, J., Petrosillo, N., Geiss, H.K., Torres, A.J. & Berger, A. (2004) Surgical site infection – a European perspective of incidence and economic burden. *International Wound Journal* **1**(4): 247–273.

Medeiros, I. & Saconato, H. (2004) Antibiotic prophylaxis for mammalian bites. In: *The Cochrane Library*, Issue 4. Chichester, John Wiley & Sons.

Moffatt, C.J., Franks, P.J., Doherty, D.C., Martin, R., Blewitt, R. & Ross, F. (2004) Prevalence of leg ulceration in a London population. *Quarterly Journal of Medicine* **97**: 431–437.

National Audit Office (2004) *Improving Emergency Care in England.* London, The Stationery Office.

National Burn Care Review Committee (2001) *Standards and Strategy for Burn Care: A Review of Burn Care in the British Isles.* London, NBCRC.

Thomas, D.R., Goode, P.S., LaMaster, K., Tennyson, T. & Parnell, L.K.S. (1999) A comparison of an opaque foam dressing versus a transparent film dressing in the management of skin tears in institutionalised subjects. *Ostomy and Wound Management* **45**(6): 22–28.

Factors that Delay Wound Healing

INTRODUCTION

Wound healing progresses through an orderly sequence, with visible signs of healing such as new granulation tissue and a reduction in wound dimensions. Although healing time varies according to the type and site of the wound, complete healing of a wound is expected to occur within an acceptable time frame. When healing of the wound fails to progress as expected or the wound deteriorates, then healing is described as delayed or impaired. Patients with a wound should be assessed, as part of their holistic assessment, for any factors that may impede healing. These will vary depending on the patient's underlying medical condition and may be missed if the focus of attention is only on dressing the wound. This chapter focuses on the main factors that adversely affect wound healing.

INFECTION

Chronic wounds are not sterile. It is widely accepted that all chronic wounds are contaminated with bacteria. A contaminated wound is considered to have non-multiplying bacteria. The healing process is not necessarily interrupted by the presence of non-multiplying bacteria. The term 'colonisation' is used to describe a chronic wound that has multiplying bacteria, without infection. The majority of chronic wounds such as pressure ulcers and leg ulcers are colonised wounds. Topical antimicrobial therapy may be considered for non-healing colonised wounds with no signs of tissue invasion (Bowler, 2001). See Chapter 4 for information on antimicrobial treatments available for treating colonised pressure ulcers and leg ulcers.

Bacteria that invade tissue and cause infection are known as 'pathogens'. The presence of infection impairs healing and reduces tensile strength. Infection is determined by clinical examination and treatment should always be with appropriate systemic antibiotic therapy (Bowler, 2001). See Chapter 5 for information on assessment of wound infection. A wound swab is taken for culture to confirm diagnosis and iden- tify the specific organisms and antibiotic sensitivities. Infected wounds tend to produce increased amounts of exudate, requiring appropriate dressings to cope with this and also more frequent dressing changes. See Chapter 4 for information on suitable dressings for heavily exuding wounds. The skin around the wound is at high risk of damage from infected wound fluid and an effective skin barrier preparation should be applied. See Chapter 6 for information on peri-wound skin care.

COMPROMISED IMMUNE SYSTEM

The immune system forms part of the body's natural defences. When the immune system is compromised all phases of healing are delayed and patients are at increased risk of infection. Those who have a compromised immune system include patients who have cancer, who are human immunodeficiency virus

(HIV)-positive, who are malnourished, and older and frail patients. The effects of some treatment can result in a compromised immune system, such as radiation therapy, chemotherapy, steroid therapy, and immuno-suppressive therapy (Stotts & Wipke-Tevis, 2001).

DIABETES

Diabetic neuropathy, peripheral vascular disease, and raised blood glucose levels (hyperglycaemia) are associated with impaired healing in patients with diabetes. Symptoms such as pain and discomfort are masked in patients with diabetic neuropathy and an initially small wound on the foot may become infected and begin discharging before the patient realises there is a problem. See Chapter 7 for information on the management of diabetic foot ulcers. Hyperglycaemia (high blood glucose) results in altered leucocyte function and increased risk of infection (Stotts & Wipke-Tevis, 2001). The inflammatory response is delayed in hyper-glycaemia, adversely affecting granulation tissue formation. Once glucose is controlled in patients with diabetes healing improves.

Decreased blood flow from atherosclerosis also has an adverse effect on wound healing. The lowered oxygen environment reduces collagen formation and increases the risk of infection (Lioupis, 2005).

MALNUTRITION

Inadequate nutrition can interfere with wound healing by delaying the healing response. It is important that a holistic assessment of the patient with a wound should include nutritional screening; patients with poor dietary intake should be referred to a dietician

(Mandal, 2006). Patients may have a low appetite while in hospital, leading to a reduction in nutritional status. Proteins, vitamins and minerals have a significant role in wound healing. Research data suggest that inadequate quantities of specific nutrients can adversely affect healing.

Protein

Patients with chronic wounds require increased levels of protein. The main protein synthesised during healing is collagen. Studies suggest that protein depletion can adversely affect wound healing, by prolonging the inflammatory phase and leading to poor collagen synthesis (Gray & Cooper, 2001). Protein deficiency and low serum albumin concentration result in oedema, reducing the passage of nutrients to damaged tissue (Baxter & Ballard, 2002).

Vitamin C

Vitamin C is important for collagen synthesis. Injury stress and sepsis increase the body's demand for vitamin C. Vitamin C deficiency results in reduced collagen deposition and increased risk of surgical wound dehiscence (Gray & Cooper, 2001).

Zinc

Patients are at risk of zinc deficiency if their food intake is decreased. Zinc is necessary for protein synthesis. Zinc deficiency results in decreased collagen synthesis and wound strength. There are conflicting data on the role of zinc in wound healing. Current evidence suggests that deficiency impairs healing and oral zinc supplementation in cases of deficiency improves the rate of healing (Wilkinson & Hawke, 1999).

There is evidence suggesting that targeting specific nutrient deficiencies may improve wound healing outcomes in pressure ulcers (Frias Soriano *et al.*, 2004).

AGEING
Wound healing and wound contraction occurs more rapidly in children than in adults and slows down significantly in older people. There is a reduction in cell proliferation as we age, and the inflammatory response occurs more slowly, collagen metabolism is reduced, angiogenesis is delayed and there is a decrease in turnover of the epidermal layer of the skin (Toy, 2005). In addition, older people often have concomitant chronic illnesses or diseases such as diabetes, cardiac disease, pulmonary disease, renal disease and cancer (Stotts & Wipke-Tevis, 2001). Most wounds in the older population eventually heal satisfactorily, although the rate of healing is much slower.

LOW OXYGEN AND DECREASED TISSUE PERFUSION
Tissue perfusion may be impaired by arterial occlusion or vasoconstriction, peripheral vascular disease, diabetes mellitus, and also as a consequence of unrelieved pressure. Pressure-relieving devices such as mattresses and cushions are available for very thin, ill, immobile or other at-risk patients. Oxygen is required for angiogenesis and the formation of collagen. Most of the oxygen content of the blood is carried

by haemoglobin; consequently patients with wounds who have low haemoglobin have impaired healing. Tobacco acts as a potent vasoconstrictor and patients who require surgery are recommended to stop smoking pre- and post-operatively (Towler, 2000).

HYPERGRANULATION

The term 'hypergranulation tissue', also referred to as over-granulation tissue, describes granulation tissue that has continued to progress above the level of the wound bed (Dunford, 1999) (Fig. 3.1). Granulation tissue fills the wound space and once it is level with the wound edges, epithelial cells migrate and proliferate from the edges or from islands within the wound bed. When hypergranulation tissue is present the raised

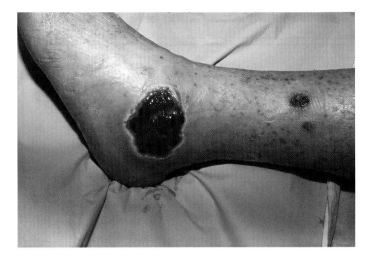

Fig. 3.1 Hypergranulation.

tissue inhibits migration of epithelial cells and healing is impaired. Hypergranulation has been reported as a common problem related to gastrostomy tubes and may also sometimes be found around tracheostomy and drain sites (Rollins, 2000). Topical steroid preparations are sometimes used to reduce and flatten hypergranulation tissue. Occlusive dressings can sometimes result in a wound becoming over-granulated. When this occurs changing from an occlusive dressing to a simple foam dressing can be helpful in reducing the hypergranulation (Harris & Rolstad, 1994). Wounds contract as they heal and in some instances hypergranulation tissue resolves by itself as the wound heals.

Key points

- Delayed or impaired healing describes a wound that fails to progress as expected or the wound deteriorates.
- Healthcare professionals need to be aware of factors that can delay wound healing to enable them to identify at risk patients.
- Infection impedes wound healing and treatment is with appropriate systemic antibiotic therapy.
- Age is an important factor as repair of damaged tissue occurs more slowly as we age.
- Nutrient deficiencies can adversely affect healing. Outcomes may be improved with specific nutritional programmes.
- Oxygen is required for angiogenesis and the formation of collagen and healing. Low levels of oxygen reduces collagen formation and increases the risk of infection.

SUMMARY

This chapter has focused on the main factors that adversely affect wound healing. You should now use the knowledge you have gained from reading this chapter to undertake the following exercise.

Exercise 3.1

Case scenario

Mr James is an elderly man aged 82 years, who lives with his daughter. His wife died 3 years ago. He has little appetite and has become quite frail and thin in the last few months. He walks very slowly with the help of a stick and spends most of his day sitting in a firm upright arm-chair. Mr James fell in the bathroom and was admitted to hospital with a fractured neck of the left femur. He has had surgery and is now 1-day post-op. He is complaining that his sacral area feels sore. On examination of the area his skin is very red but intact.

Using a systematic approach, identify the relevant factors that might impact on the healing process of this patient's surgical wound and pressure ulcer.

Step 1: assess the patient, wound and circumstances
Mr James is frail and thin, with a surgical wound on his left hip and he is also at risk of developing a sacral pressure ulcer. In his assessment you need to consider whether he is malnourished and his level of mobility.

Continued

Step 2: utilise existing information about the patient
You should consider whether Mr James' diet has been inadequate and whether he needs a nutritional supplement. Following assessment of his mobility you need to consider how much help Mr James will require to get him fully mobile again and who else will be involved in this. You already know that Mr James spends a great deal of time sitting down. He is also relatively immobile following surgery. You should consider what type of seating and mattress would be appropriate for him.

Step 3: explore relevant current best practice
Consider what nutritional supplements are available on the ward for the patients. You need to determine where suitable seating and mattress aids are available in the area you are working. You need to follow the protocol for your area regarding mobility following hip surgery.

Step 4: make a clinical decision
You should have enough information to identify potential factors that could impede Mr James' wound healing and recovery and prevent tissue breakdown in his sacral area. Write these down and think about how they can be resolved. The factors should include his dietary needs, his mobility needs and any requirements for suitable seating.

Step 5: evaluate progress
Evaluation of the patient's care and progress should include evidence of a clean healthy healing surgical wound. There should be a noticeable improvement in his diet and he should achieve an accepted level of mobility for his age and condition.

Suggested management

The goal is for this patient's surgical wound to heal without complications and maintenance of skin integrity in his sacral area. Mr James has become very thin recently and has little appetite and should be referred to a dietician, as he will require additional nutritional support. Inadequate nutrition can interfere with wound healing by delaying the healing response. Many liquid nutritional supplements are available, and they are used in conjunction with normal food. Mr James is very thin and will require a pressure-relieving cushion in his chair and a pressure-relieving mattress. Pressure-relieving aids are sometimes available on the ward or can be requested through the relevant department in the hospital. Mr James will need to have physiotherapy to help him regain his mobility following surgery. He should be encouraged to follow the exercises given to him by the physiotherapist.

CONCLUSION

This exercise has shown you how to work through the decision-making process in a systematic way to enable you to identify the relevant factors that might impact on the healing process of Mr James' surgical wound and prevent him having a pressure ulcer.

REFERENCES

Baxter, H. & Ballard, K. (2002) Delayed wound healing. *Clinical Education in Wound Management Booklet.* Holsworthy, Medical Communications.

Bowler, P. (2001) The role of bacteria in wound healing: research or myth. In: Oxford Wound Healing Institute. *The Oxford Wound Healing Course Handbook.* Oxford, Positif Press.

Dunford, C. (1999) Hypergranulation tissue. *Journal of Wound Care* **8**(10): 506–507.

Frias Soriano, L., Lage Vazquez, M.A., Perez-Potabella Mristany, C., Xandri Graupera, Wouters-Wesseling, W. & Wagenaar, L. (2004) The effectiveness of oral nutritional supplementation in the healing of pressure ulcers. *Journal of Wound Care* **13**(8): 319–322.

Gray, D. & Cooper, P. (2001) Nutrition and healing: what is the link? *Journal of Wound Care* **10**(3): 86–89.

Harris, A. & Rolstad, B.S. (1994) Hypergranulation tissue: a non traumatic method of management. *Ostomy and Wound Management* **40**(5): 20–30.

Lioupis, C. (2005) Effects of diabetes on wound healing: an update. *Journal of Wound Care* **14**(2): 84–86.

Mandal, A. (2006) Do malnutrition and nutritional supplementation have an effect on the wound healing process. *Journal of Wound Care* **15**(6): 254–257.

Rollins, H. (2000) Hypergranulation tissue at gastrostomy sites. *Journal of Wound Care* **9**(3):127–129.

Stotts, N.A. & Wipke-Tevis, D.D. (2001) Co-factors in impaired wound healing. In: Krasner, D.L., Rodeheaver, G.T. & Sibbald, R.G. (eds) *Chronic Wound Care: A Clinical Source Book for Healthcare Professionals, Third Edition.* Wayne, PA, H.M.P. Communications, pp. 265–272.

Towler, J. (2000) Cigarette smoking and its effects on wound healing. *Journal of Wound Care* **9**(3): 100–104.

Toy, L.W. (2005) How much do we understand about the effects of aging on healing? *Journal of Wound Care* **14**(10): 472–476.

Wilkinson, E. & Hawke, C. (1999) Zinc and chronic leg ulcers: a systematic review of oral zinc in the treatment of leg ulcers. *Journal of Tissue Viability* **9**(1): 21.

General Principles of Wound Management

4

INTRODUCTION

Nurses are predominantly the healthcare professionals with responsibility for the application of wound dressings. All nurses undertaking dressing change have a duty to their patients to provide care that is safe, effective and as comfortable as possible. This chapter will consider the basic principles of asepsis relevant to wound care and how to change a dressing. Some of the dressings in general use will also be described. This is intended to be a very practical chapter, but it should be read alongside chapters such as Chapter 5, which looks at assessment and planning, and Chapter 7, which provides guidance on the management of specific types of wound.

BASIC PRINCIPLES OF ASEPSIS IN WOUND MANAGEMENT

Asepsis literally means the absence of harmful bacteria and is the term used to describe prevention of contamination of body tissues by either killing or removing micro-organisms (Xavier, 1999). Dressing change is often referred to as an 'aseptic technique', which means that items coming in contact with a wound are sterile and the techniques used specifically aim to prevent the spread of infection into the wound. Thus all dressings and dressing packs are placed in individual sealed packs and sterilised during the manu-facturing process and sterile gloves are worn during the procedure.

Attention to effective hand washing is an essential part of the procedure. In fact hand hygiene is seen as so important that it is one of the four standard principles in the national guidelines for preventing infections in hospitals (Pratt *et al.*, 2007). The guidelines state that hands should be washed with either soap and water or an alcohol-based handrub ensuring that every part of the hands is cleansed. Figure 4.1 shows the preferred hand cleansing technique based on Taylor's recom-mendations which can be used with either method of hand washing (Taylor, 1978). Areas that are often missed are the areas between the fingers, the tips of the fingers and the thumbs. When using soap and water the soap should be rinsed off and the hands dried thoroughly. In a review of the literature to investigate the impact of the use of soap and water and alcohol-based handrubs on levels of skin irritation, Pellowe *et al.* (2003) concluded that these products were poten-tially damaging to skin. Therefore, the national guide-lines recommend the regular use of skin emollient creams to assist in maintaining skin integrity (Pratt *et al.*, 2007).

It should also be noted that all jewellery should be removed, including bracelets, necklaces and watches. Rings with stones should be removed and only a plain metal ring such as a wedding ring may be worn. Fin-gernails should be kept short and without nail polish and false nails and nail extensions should not be worn in the clinical area (Pratt *et al.*, 2007). Hair should be securely tied back from the face and long hair should

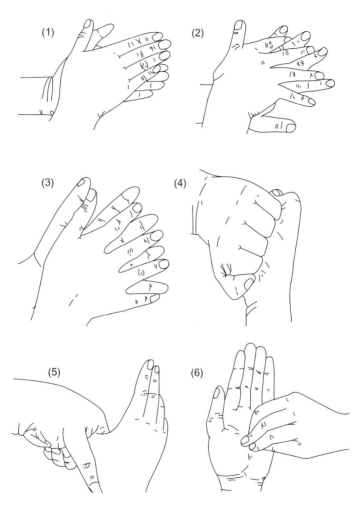

Fig. 4.1 Hand washing technique.

be tied. It is an infection control hazard to have hair or jewellery dangling over a wound. It also looks unprofessional and most patients will find it a cause for concern. Hospitals have a uniform policy and expect nurses to have removed jewellery and tied their hair back before coming on duty.

There has been some debate about whether an aseptic technique is necessary for dressing changes in chronic wounds, especially as a certain amount of ritual has been associated with it in the past (Hollinworth & Kingston, 1998). After reviewing the topic, Gilmour (2000) concluded that, despite the amount of ritual associated with aseptic technique, it remains an effective strategy to prevent cross-infection. The difference between a clean and an aseptic technique is that clean single-use gloves rather than sterile gloves are worn and tap water may be used to clean the wound. All remaining items such as dressings and dressing packs are sterile. The procedure should be undertaken in the same way whether it is an aseptic or a clean procedure as cross-infection remains a hazard and chronic wounds are just as vulnerable to infection as any other type of wound.

CHANGING A DRESSING

Dressing changes should be undertaken in a systematic way. The five-step systematic approach can be utilised to undertake the procedure.

Step 1: assess the patient, wound and circumstances

It is important to read the wound care plan before preparing any equipment. The plan should provide information about the type of wound, its appearance when last assessed, the dressing being used and any adjunctive treatment. This information is essential when assembling the necessary equipment to change the dressing. In addition, the nurse should communicate with the patient and ensure that timing of the dressing change does not conflict with any other aspect of care or activity. For example, if a patient has to visit the physiotherapy department, it makes sense for the dressing change to be undertaken beforehand. However, if the patient wishes to have a shower, then it would be best to change the dressing immediately afterwards.

Step 2: utilise existing information about the patient

The plan of care should indicate whether or not dressing changes have been particularly painful for the patient in the past and what methods have been used to alleviate the pain. Should the patient require analgesia, it must be given to the patient and sufficient time allowed for it to become effective before the dressing procedure commences. For more information about wound pain, see Chapter 8.

Step 3: explore relevant current best practice

This step involves applying current best practice to the procedure.

- Wash your hands carefully and dry them thoroughly. Put on a clean plastic apron.
- Clean the trolley to be used by spraying with alcohol spray and allow to dry for 1 minute. Any excess

alcohol may then be mopped up with a paper towel.

• Assemble all the items needed for the procedure, which may include a dressing pack, gauze swabs, the new dressing, sterile saline, strapping or bandages, and place them on the bottom shelf of the trolley.

• Ensure patient privacy by closing the curtains and prepare the patient by placing them in the best position to get clear access to the wound, while maintaining patient comfort. This may be in a bed or a chair or a couch in a treatment room. Remove relevant clothing and bedclothes, always being careful to maintain patient dignity, to ensure a clear area around the wound. Loosen the outer strapping of the old dressing.

• Wash hands with soap and water and dry thoroughly, or cleanse thoroughly with alcohol-based handrub.

• Ensuring that the dressing pack is intact and dry, open the outer bag at one end and slide out the contents onto the top shelf of the trolley. Using finger tips only, pull open the four corners of the inner wrapping to cover the top of the trolley and form a sterile field from which to work (see Fig. 4.2). Prepare any strips of strapping that may be required and attach to the side of the trolley or open bandages and place to the side of the patient.

• Clean hands thoroughly with alcohol-based handrub.

• Add any other dressings required by opening outer wrapping and dropping on to the sterile field without touching the contents. The items on the sterile field

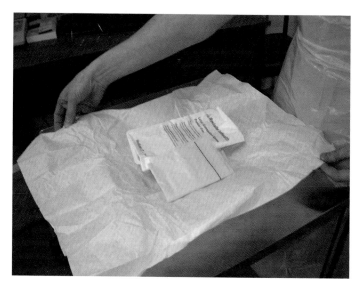

Fig. 4.2 Opening the dressing pack.

can be rearranged by picking up the waste disposable bag included in the dressing pack, inserting a hand into it and then using it to rearrange the items as required (Figs 4.3 and 4.4).

- Keeping this hand inside the disposable bag, the used dressing can be removed. Then the bag should be inverted so that the dirty dressing is inside the bag. The tape on the bag should then be removed to allow the sticky edge of the bag to be stuck to the edge of the trolley so that it is ready to receive any further waste items.
- Clean hands thoroughly with alcohol-based handrub.

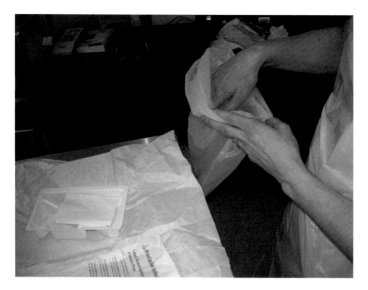

Fig. 4.3 Inserting hand into yellow disposal bag.

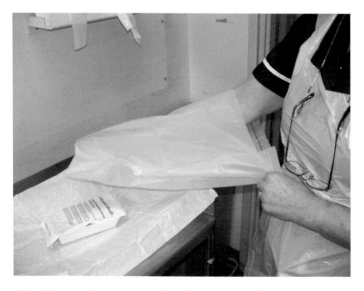

Fig. 4.4 Using bag-covered hand to rearrange items on dressing trolley.

- Put on the sterile gloves included in the dressing pack, ensuring that only the inner side of the gloves is touched.
- Clean the wound, if necessary, using either gauze moistened in saline or a syringe filled with saline to remove remnants of the old dressing, dried exudate, loose slough or loose skin scales. Gently dry the skin around the wound with a clean gauze swab.
- Apply the new dressing and secure appropriately.
- Remove gloves and fold up all remaining items in the sterile field and place inside disposable bag.
- Help the patient to replace any garments as required, and make them comfortable.
- Remove trolley and dispose the waste bag into a yellow clinical waste bag.
- Clean the trolley as before and return it to its usual storage place.
- Remove apron and wash hands thoroughly in soap and water.

Step 4: make a clinical decision

During the process of changing a dressing it is important to assess the wound carefully. This starts with looking at the outer side of the dressing before it is removed to see if there are signs of exudate leakage. It is also useful to discover from the patient when the dressing was last changed. If the dressing is leaking then it may require changing more frequently than stated in the care plan. Once the old dressing has been removed and the wound cleansed, the wound appearance should be assessed for any changes since the previous assessment. (Wound assessment is covered in detail in Chapter 5.) If the appearance differs greatly then a change of plan may be indicated. If there are signs of infection or a reaction to the dressing, it is advisable to get further advice from the nurse in charge or a doctor.

Step 5: evaluate progress

The final step is to record that a dressing change has been undertaken. This should include details of the wound assessment, any measurements that may have been taken and whether any changes have been made to the existing wound care plan.

DIFFERENT TYPES OF DRESSING

There are many different dressings available and it can seem extremely bewildering when selecting an appropriate dressing. Careful assessment of the wound, as discussed in Chapter 5, is essential before making a decision. This section is intended to provide the reader with some understanding of the range of dressings commonly used in practice and examples of brand names in each category of dressing are given in Table 4.1. More detailed information about the full range of wound management products can be found in Dealey (2005) and at www.dressings.org.

Gauze products

Gauze swabs have been used for many years in wound care, both as a primary dressing in direct contact with the wound and as a secondary dressing over a primary dressing. They have a number of disadvantages: they stick to the wound and can be painful to remove, damaging new tissue; and they have little absorbency and exudate can easily soak through, creating a potential

Table 4.1 Examples of different types of dressings.

Type of dressing	Brand names	Manufacturer
Non-adherent dressings	Adaptic	Johnson & Johnson Medical Ltd
	Melolin	Smith & Nephew Healthcare Ltd
	NA Dressings	Johnson & Johnson Medical Ltd
	Telfa	The Kendall Company Ltd
Alginates	Algisite M	Smith & Nephew Healthcare Ltd
	Kaltostat	ConvaTec Ltd
	Seasorb Soft	Coloplast Ltd
	Sorbsan	Unomedical Ltd
	Tegaderm Alginate Dressing	3M UK Plc
Films	Cutifilm	Smith & Nephew Healthcare Ltd
	Opsite	Smith & Nephew Healthcare Ltd
	Tegaderm Film Dressing	3M UK Plc
Foams	Allevyn	Smith & Nephew Healthcare Ltd
	Tegaderm Foam Dressing	3M UK Plc
	Tielle	Johnson & Johnson Medical Ltd
Foams (combination)	UrgoCell	Urgo Laboratories
	Versiva	ConvaTec Ltd

Continued

Table 4.1 *Continued*

Type of dressing	Brand names	Manufacturer
Hydrocolloids	Comfeel Plus	Coloplast Ltd
	Duoderm	ConvaTec Ltd
	Granuflex	ConvaTec Ltd
	Tegaderm Hydrocolloid Dressing	3M UK Plc
Hydrogels	Actiform Cool	Activa Healthcare Ltd
	Intrasite	Smith & Nephew Healthcare Ltd
	Nu-Gel	Johnson & Johnson Medical Ltd
	Purilon	Coloplast Ltd
Silicone dressings	Biobrane	Smith & Nephew Healthcare Ltd
	Cica-Care	Smith & Nephew Healthcare Ltd
	Mepiform	Mölnlycke Health Care
	Mepilex	Mölnlycke Health Care
	Mepitel	Mölnlycke Health Care
Silver dressings	Acticoat	Smith & Nephew Healthcare Ltd
	Actisorb Silver 220	Johnson & Johnson Medical Ltd
	Aquacel Ag	ConvaTec Ltd
	Contreet	Coloplast Ltd
	UrgoCell Silver	Urgo Laboratories
Honey dressings	Activon Tulle	Advancis Medical
	Algivon	Advancis Medical
	Medihoney	Medihoney Pty
	Mesitran	Unomedical Ltd

route for bacteria to penetrate through to the wound. They have little place as a primary dressing for open wounds.

Absorbent pads are a variation on gauze and generally made of synthetic materials with additional absorbent materials stitched inside. They can be a very useful secondary dressing as they can assist in absorbing exudate. They are available in a range of sizes and are cheap. Both absorbent pads and gauze swabs require some form of strapping to hold them in place.

Low adherent dressings

These dressings are an improvement on gauze as they are less likely to adhere to the wound. They vary slightly in structure depending on the brand, but generally comprise a thin perforated plastic wound contact layer, a thin central core of absorbent fibres and an outer layer, which is a non-woven fabric or a continuation of the inner layer. Care should be given to ensure that the dressing is applied with the wound contact layer next to the wound or the dressing will stick like gauze. These dressings have little absorbency and may require a secondary pad. They require strapping or bandages to hold them in place.

A variation of the low adherent dressings is the island dressing. These dressings have a central pad covered with an adhesive fabric. They come in a range of sizes and can conform to awkward areas of the body. They are useful for wounds with low levels of exudate. Remember that the central pad needs to cover the wound when determining the correct size to use.

Alginates

Alginates are described as interactive dressings, which means that they change their structure when they come in contact with the wound fluid. Alginate dressings are made from various formulations of seaweed, depending on the brand, and look like a thin fibrous sheet. They are also available in a rope format for use in cavity wounds. As the alginate dressing absorbs exudate, the fibres soften and form a gel. These dressings are very absorbent and can be used on heavily exuding wounds. They are not suitable for low exuding wounds as they can stick to the wound. When changing the dressing ensure that all of the used dressing is removed as it can form a crust around the wound. It is important to follow the manufacturer's instructions for application and removal. Some brands can be removed as one sheet after moistening with normal saline while others may need irrigation with normal saline to flush out the old dressing. Alginates do not need to overlap the wound edges and require a secondary dressing such as an absorbent pad which needs taping in place.

Films

Film dressings are made from a thin layer of polyurethane with an adhesive coating. The dressing is semi-permeable, in other words, oxygen and water vapour can pass through it, but bacteria cannot penetrate the film. The dressing does not have any absorbency and is not suitable for wounds with moderate to high levels of exudate. When selecting an appropriate size of dressing allow for a 4–5 cm overlap onto the surrounding skin.

Film dressings have some type of carrier to prevent the film wrinkling during the application process. However, the type of carrier varies depending on the manufacturer. No secondary dressing is required with a film dressing. Care should be taken if using the dressing on wounds surrounded by fragile skin as the adhesive can damage the skin when the dressing is removed. The dressing should be removed by lifting a corner of the film and gently stretching it away from the centre of the film to break the adhesion. This process is repeated until all the dressing has lifted from the wound. On no account should the dressing be pulled off the skin without stretching the film first, as this can cause trauma to the skin and unnecessary pain to the patient.

Foams

Foam dressings are made from polyurethane foam and generally have a waterproof backing. There is some variation in the layers of the dressing depending on the manufacturer. Some foam dressings have an adhesive border and others require to be held in place with tape or bandages, and all require some overlap over the wound edges ranging from 2 cm to 5 cm. Foam dressings generally have good absorptive capacity, and they are useful on wounds with moderate to heavy exudate.

Hydrocolloids

Hydrocolloid dressings are generally made from a polyurethane film with an adhesive mass attached to it to form a flexible wafer. The components of the adhesive mass vary according to the manufacturer, but common components are pectin and sodium carboxymethylcellulose. Hydrocolloids are also a type of interactive dressing, and as they absorb exudate, the adhesive mass swells and forms a gel with a distinctive odour. They are best used on wounds with moderate to low levels of exudate. There are many varieties of hydrocolloid dressings, all of which require slightly different methods of application and may or may not require a secondary dressing. All manufacturers are required to provide instructions on application with their products and they can be useful in ensuring effective application.

Hydrogels

Hydrogels are an aqueous gel made from different materials depending on the brand. They are also interactive dressings as the gel becomes liquid as it absorbs exudate. Hydrogels are able to donate moisture to the wound which assists in hydrating any slough or eschar and promotes autolysis. Most hydrogels have some type of applicator which allows the gel to be squeezed into the wound. They require a secondary dressing such as an absorbent pad and are best used on wounds with low to moderate exudate.

Iodine-based dressings

Iodine is a widely used antiseptic. It can be found in several different formats. There are two dressings using cadexomer-iodine. One comes in a gel format which can be squeezed into the wound, in the other version the cadexomer iodine is impregnated into a pad that is laid onto the wound. Both these dressings are absorbent and promote debridement as well as having an antimicrobial effect. A rather different type of dressing comprises a low adherent dressing impregnated with povidone iodine. The dressing is not absorbent and is mostly used on minor traumatic injuries. Iodine dressings should not be used for long periods of time because the iodine can be absorbed by the thyroid gland.

Silicone dressings
Silicone dressings are made from soft polymers and have a slightly tacky wound contact layer. This means that they can be removed without causing any trauma to the wound or surrounding skin. There are several different types of silicone dressing. The silicone wound contact layer has a variety of different backings which impact on the level of absorbency and the overall purpose of the dressing. For example, one type of silicone dressing has three layers: an outer vapour-permeable polyurethane membrane, a polyurethane foam central layer providing absorbency and a soft silicone wound contact layer.

Silver dressings
Silver is considered to be a useful antimicrobial and is available in a variety of different formats. Silver in the form of a silver sulphadiazine cream has been used for many years in the management of burns. More recently, silver has been seen to be effective in treating wounds infected with methicillin-resistant *Staphylococcus aureus* (MRSA) and there has been considerable interest in its use. As a result silver-coated dressings and dressings to which silver has been added such as foams and hydrocolloids, are available.

Honey-based dressings

Honey has been used to treat wounds for many centuries and has recently become popular again. However, not all types of honey are suitable; Manuka honey from New Zealand is recognised as the most appropriate for use in wound care. Honey has an antimicrobial effect and can absorb exudate, but it is also quite sticky and requires careful application. Honey is available in a tube or added to other dressings such as a synthetic mesh or alginates.

Other wound management therapies

Generally the dressings described above can be applied easily following a little training. However, some therapies such as biosurgery or topical negative-pressure therapy require greater levels of competence and specialist knowledge in their use.

Biosurgery

Biosurgery is also known as larvae or maggot therapy. Sterile maggots are applied to necrotic, infected or sloughy wounds where they liquefy the slough and necrotic tissue and ingest it. Maggots require moisture in order to become active and so should not be used on wounds with a necrotic eschar. Careful application and removal is necessary to ensure that the surrounding skin is protected, the maggots have the correct environment in which to work and that they do not escape from the wound.

Topical negative pressure therapy (TNP)

TNP is also sometimes referred to vacuum-assisted closure (VAC). It comprises a foam sponge which is connected to a pump and canister by a tube. The sponge is cut to the shape of the wound and the tube inserted into it. This is then covered by a plastic adhesive film to seal the wound and assist in creating a vacuum when the pump is turned on. The pump exerts a low pressure on the wound and draws exudate into the canister. TNP is used in a variety of situations to control heavy exudate, the debridement of sloughy or infected wounds and to promote granulation.

METHODS OF DRESSING RETENTION

The main methods of retaining dressings are the use of surgical tapes and bandages.

Surgical tapes

Surgical tapes or strapping are generally made from some type of non-woven fabric with an adhesive coating. Although modern tapes are mainly hypo-allergenic, in some patients they can still cause skin irritation. They are available in several widths and some have a slight ability to stretch, which is useful when applying over joints. Some tapes can easily be torn into strips whereas others need to be cut with scissors. Strapping should always be applied in such a way that all the edges of the dressing are sealed down securely.

Bandages

Many types of bandages are available, which can be used for a variety of purposes such as using a support bandage for a sprained ankle. This is too big a topic to be covered here and only simple bandages to retain dressings will be discussed. Retention bandages are made from cotton or non-woven fabric and have little or no elasticity. They are available in a bandage or tubular bandage format and can be found in various widths. Only sufficient length of bandage necessary to secure the dressing need be applied and care should be taken to ensure that it is not applied too tightly.

Key points

- Nurses need to understand the basic principles of asepsis before they can safely undertake a dressing change.
- Dressing change needs to be undertaken in a systematic way.
- Effective hand washing is an essential aspect of dressing change.
- There is a very wide range of dressings available and selection should only be made following a careful assessment of the wound.

SUMMARY

This chapter has discussed the issues regarding changing a wound dressing and some of the common types of wound management products. It is meant to be read in conjunction with Chapter 5 which covers assessing wounds and developing a plan of care.

You should now use the knowledge you have gained from reading this chapter to undertake the following exercise.

Exercise 4.1

Case scenario

Hilda Greenwood is a 54-year-old woman who has an abdominal wound following a hysterectomy. Her wound is healing well and she is finding her current dressing very comfortable. However, she is a large lady and has found standing up straight and walking difficult since the operation. Hilda has been having some physiotherapy and is using a walking frame to get about. She is able to get in and out of her bed with a little help. Due to her size, Hilda finds it difficult to breathe if she lies too flat in bed and prefers to sleep propped up with four to five pillows. Hilda is due for discharge after lunch and is due to have her dressing changed beforehand. You have been asked to prepare a trolley ready for her to have her dressing changed and to take her to the treatment room and make her comfortable. The couches in the treatment room are hydraulic and can be lowered for the patient to get on, then raised again for the dressing procedure. Hilda's primary nurse is going to undertake the dressing and you can stay with her and observe the dressing change.

Using a systematic approach identify the needs of this patient when preparing for their dressing change procedure.

Step 1: assess the patient, wound and circumstances
Consider what you will tell this patient about the dressing change procedure. What considerations should you give the patient? Think about when you are going to prepare the trolley and what you should do first. You need to consider how mobile Hilda is and how you will move her

Continued

from the bed to the treatment room. You will also need to consider what help she might require to get on to the couch and how you will make Hilda comfortable for her dressing to be changed.

Step 2: utilise existing information about the patient
You already know that Hilda's wound is healing and that she is happy with her current dressing. Think about how you will establish which necessary equipment you will need for the dressing change.

Step 3: explore relevant current best practice
Read step 3 again in the section 'Changing a dressing' in this chapter and consider what you should do to maintain a safe environment when preparing the dressing trolley.

Step 4: make a clinical decision
You need to consider how you will monitor that Hilda is comfortable at all times when you move her from her bed to the treatment room and get her ready for her dressing to be changed.

Step 5: evaluate progress
You should consider how you would evaluate that Hilda is in a comfortable and appropriate position for her dressing to be changed.

Suggested management
Good patient communication is essential and the first consideration should be to establish the patient's needs. The procedure should be explained to the patient and they should be encouraged to ask any questions and given time to prepare themselves. Although Hilda can

walk well with a frame she may find the distance to the treatment room too far and require a wheelchair. The wound care plan should always be consulted to identify materials required for the dressing change and the dressing trolley prepared before moving the patient.

Current best practice should be applied to the procedure. This involves washing your hands, putting on a clean plastic apron and spraying the trolley with an appropriate alcohol spray. All items required for the dressing change should be assembled and placed on the lower shelf of the trolley. You already know that Hilda's wound is healing well and that she is comfortable with her current dressing. Therefore the dressing materials can be assembled as for her previous dressing. This includes a dressing pack, gauze swabs, the new dressing and sterile saline.

When the trolley is ready Hilda can be taken to the treatment room. As Hilda is able to get on to her bed with little help and the couch can be lowered she should be able to get onto the couch with the same amount of help. You already know that Hilda is unable to lie flat and likes to be propped up in bed. Therefore you should have enough pillows for Hilda to be comfortable while she has her dressing changed. You should ask her if she is comfortable once settled on the couch and for her to inform you if she is uncomfortable at any time. You should continue to observe her throughout the dressing change for any signs of anxiety or distress due to discomfort in her position.

CONCLUSION

This exercise has shown you how to use a systematic approach to enable you to identify the needs of the patient when preparing for a dressing change procedure.

REFERENCES

Dealey, C. (2005) *The Care of Wounds, Third Edition.* Oxford, Blackwell Science.

Gilmour, D. (2000) Is aseptic technique always necessary? *Journal of Community Nursing* **14**(4): 32–35.

Hollinworth, H. & Kingston, J. (1998) Using a non-sterile technique in wound care. *Professional Nurse* **13**(4): 226–229.

Pellowe, C.M., Pratt, R.J., Harper, P., Loveday, H.P., Robinson, N., Jones, S.R.L.J. & MacRae, E.D. The Guideline Development Group: Mulhall, A., Smith, G.W., Bray, J., Carroll, A., Chieveley Williams, S., Colpman, D., Cooper, L., McInnes, E., McQuarrie, I., Newey, J., Peters, J., Pratelli, N., Richardson, G., Shah, P.J.R., Silk, D. & Wheatley, C. (2003) Evidence-based guidelines for preventing healthcare-associated infections in primary and community care in England. *Journal of Hospital Infection* **55**(suppl)(2): S1–127.

Pratt, R.J., Pellowe, C.M., Wilson, J.A., Loveday, H.P., Harper, P.J., Jones, S.R.L.J., McDougall, C. & Wilcox, M.H. (2007) Epic2: national evidence-based guidelines for preventing healthcare-associated infections in NHS hospitals in England. *Journal of Hospital Infection* **65**(suppl)(1): S1–64.

Taylor, L.J. (1978) An evaluation of hand washing techniques parts 1 & 2. *Nursing Times* **74**(2): 54 and **74**(3): 108–110.

Xavier, G. (1999) Asepsis. *Nursing Standard* **13**(36): 49–53.

Assessment, Planning and Documentation

5

INTRODUCTION

Like any other aspect of nursing care, careful assessment is essential for the provision of good wound care. This chapter describes the assessment process of a patient with a wound, using a step-by-step guide that explores what the assessment process involves and how the process develops into a plan of care to promote healing and improve the patient's quality of life. The term 'holistic' assessment is used to describe a plan of care that has been drawn up following an assessment that focuses on the patient as well as the wound. It is therefore important to read this chapter in conjunction with Chapter 3, which looks at specific factors associated with the patient that might affect wound healing. This chapter describes how to assess wounds so that an effective plan of care can be established. In addition, the importance of clear documentation is discussed. Examples of assessment forms that can be used in your own clinical practice are included.

ASSESSMENT

Wound assessment can be simplified by dividing the process into a number of questions:

- What type of wound is it?
- Where is it on the body?
- What does the wound look like?
- What is the surrounding skin like?

Each one of these questions will be addressed in turn.

What type of wound is it?

Part of the assessment should include identifying the underlying cause or aetiology of the wound. The various types of wound are described in Chapter 2. However, it is important to identify the cause of a wound, as the patient may require additional treatments, affecting their plan of care. For example, if a patient has a skin laceration it could have been caused by a fall or as a result of an animal bite. If the latter is the case then the patient is likely to require antibiotics because of the high risk of infection, whereas if it was the result of a simple fall, antibiotics are generally unnecessary. Details of the assessment and management of specific types of wound are given in Chapter 7.

Where is it on the body?

It is important to describe the anatomical position of a wound for several reasons:

- It may be useful in determining the underlying aetiology. For example if a person with diabetes has an ulcer on the sole of their foot, it is most likely to have a different cause than an ulcer on the ankle. If a patient has several wounds in different places on their body, it is important to differentiate between them, as they may have different aetiologies.

- The position of a wound may affect dressing choice. For example, although most dressings are easy to retain on a wound on the arm, it can be more problematic if a wound is on the heel or over a joint.

What does the wound look like?

Assessing wound appearance takes both skill and experience and it obviously takes time to acquire both. However, there are some basic principles that can be applied. Wounds may be open or closed. Open wounds are wounds such as leg ulcers or pressure ulcers where the skin edges are separated, whereas in closed wounds the skin edges are held together. Examples of closed wounds are surgical wounds where the skin edges are held together with sutures or clips and lacerations where there is no skin loss. As well as determining the shape and size of a wound, the wound bed of open wounds must also be assessed. Assessment of the wound bed together with the amount and colour of any exudate present is important as it allows the healthcare professional to determine the status of the wound: whether it is healing or static and if there are any signs of complications such as infection. Increased levels of exudate production may be associated with high bacterial growth in the wound. Normal wound exudate has a pale straw colour, but it may become discoloured and viscous (thick) in the presence of infection (Cutting & White, 2002). The amount of wound exudate may be determined by assessing the interaction with the dressing (as shown in Table 5.1) (World Union of Wound Healing Societies, 2007). Generally,

Table 5.1 Evaluation of dressing: exudate interaction.

Status	Indicators
Dry	Wound bed is dry: there is no visible moisture and the primary dressing is unmarked; dressing may adhere to the wound. **NB**: This may be the environment of choice for ischaemic wounds.
Moist	Small amounts of fluid are visible when the dressing is removed; the primary dressing may be lightly marked; dressing frequency change is appropriate for the dressing type. **NB**: In many cases, this is the aim of exudate management.
Wet	Small amounts of fluid are visible when the dressing is removed; the primary dressing is extensively marked, but strikethrough is not occurring; dressing frequency change is appropriate for the dressing type.
Saturated	Primary dressing is wet and strikethrough is occurring; dressing change is required more frequently than usual for the dressing type; periwound skin may be macerated.
Leaking	Dressings are saturated and exudate is escaping from primary and secondary dressings onto clothes or beyond; dressing change is required much more frequently than usual for dressing type.

Reproduced by kind permission from World Healing Societies. *Principles of Best Practice: Wound Exudates and the Role of Dressings. A Consensus Document.* London, MEP Ltd, 2007. © MEP Ltd 2007.

wounds are described as necrotic, infected, sloughy, granulating or epithelialising. Each one of these categories will now be described including the level and type of exudate associated with each category.

Necrotic wounds

Necrotic wounds are wounds either covered in dead tissue like a black leathery scab known as eschar or with a black or brown slough in the base of the wound. Fig. 5.1 shows two wounds, one covered with a necrotic eschar and the other with necrotic slough filling the wound bed. There is no exudate with necrotic eschar, but necrotic slough has a highly offensive, often copious, exudate.

Treatment aim: Necrotic tissue has to be removed from a wound to allow it to heal. This is often called debridement.

Infected wounds

Just as we all have bacteria on our skin, all wounds will have some bacteria on the surface. However, if the levels of bacteria or the virulence of the bacteria increase beyond the body's ability to resist, then infection will occur. Often the first indication of infection is increased pain in the wound. There is usually also increased exudate, which may have a particular colour or odour depending on the bacteria causing the infection. The skin around the wound may be red and warm to touch. The infection spreads into the surrounding tissues, especially subcutaneous tissue; this is known as cellulitis. Cellulitis is a serious condition that is very painful for the patient and requires intensive antibiotics and possible hospitalisation.

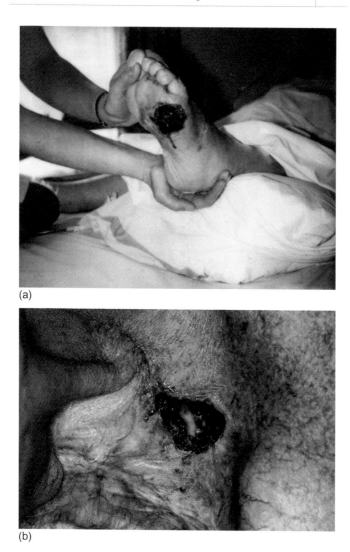

Fig. 5.1 Necrotic wounds showing necrotic eschar (a) and necrotic slough (b).

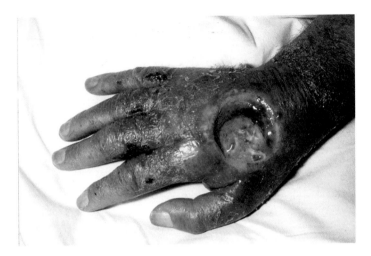

Fig. 5.2 An infected wound.

Fig. 5.2 shows an infected wound where there is no extension of the infection beyond the wound area. Compare it with Fig. 5.3, which shows a clearly cellulitic leg, where infection has spread into the tissues causing extensive erythema, swelling and induration.

Aim of treatment: The aim here is to treat the infection and prevent spread of the infection elsewhere in the body.

Sloughy wounds

Cells involved in the healing process, such as neutrophils and macrophages, only live for short periods. The dead cells form a creamy coloured fairly thin slough on the wound bed. At this stage of a wound's progress the exudate is usually moderate to heavy in quantity.

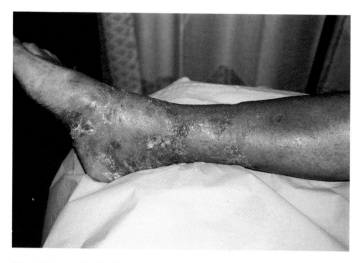

Fig. 5.3 A cellulitic leg.

This type of slough is part of normal wound healing as discussed in Chapter 1, unlike the type of slough previously described in necrotic and infected wounds. Fig. 5.4 shows this type of slough in a leg ulcer and illustrates how much thinner it is than in necrotic and infected wounds. As the slough resolves, granulation tissue will start to be seen in the wound bed.

Aim of treatment: To provide a moist environment on the wound surface which will promote the natural progression of the wound towards healing.

Granulating wounds
As an open wound heals the wound bed becomes filled with red granulation tissue. It has a granular or knobbly appearance, as shown in Fig. 5.5, caused by

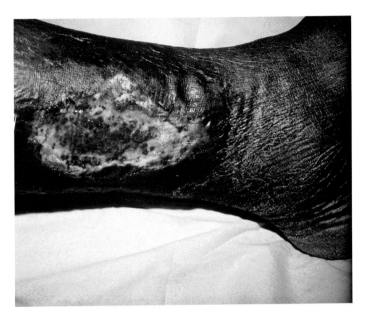

Fig. 5.4 A sloughy wound.

capillary loops projecting higher than the scaffolding matrix supporting them. As the wound bed fills with new tissue, the level of exudate gradually reduces.

Aim of treatment: To protect the newly formed, fragile tissue in the wound bed from any damage and encourage it to continue to heal.

Epithelialising wounds

Once the wound bed is filled with granulation tissue the cells round the wound margin start to divide forming a slight pink-coloured ridge. As the new cells

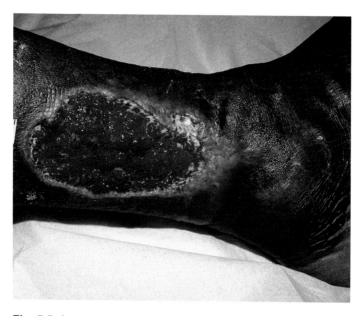

Fig. 5.5 A granulating wound.

spread across the wound surface it is easy to see the process of epithelialisation because of the white/pink colour of the new tissue. It is important to note that all epithelial tissue is initially white/pink regardless of the colour of the patient's skin and it only regains its normal hue as normal pigmentation returns after a few weeks. There is now little or no exudate and the new tissue is quite fragile. Fig. 5.6 shows a wound which is partially covered in epithelial tissue. It is possible to see the slightly irregular way in which the cells cover the wound surface.

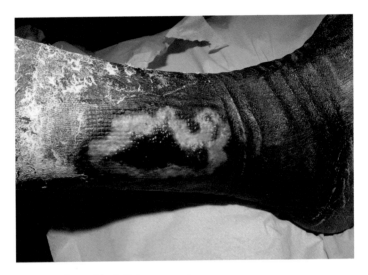

Fig. 5.6 An epithelialising wound.

Aim of treatment: To protect the wound and encourage it to continue to heal.

What is the surrounding skin like?

The final aspect of the assessment process is to consider the status of the skin surrounding the wound. It may be an indicator of the state of the wound, for example becoming red and hot in the presence of infection, or it may need special protection if there is heavy wound exudate causing the skin to become macerated. More information about peri-wound skin is given in Chapter 6.

MEASURING WOUND SIZE

It is very useful to measure a wound in order to monitor its progress. A number of different methods can be used, which will vary among clinical areas. The simplest method of measuring a wound is to draw a small sketch of its shape on the assessment chart and measure the greatest length and the greatest width, marking the points of measurement on the sketch (Fig. 5.7). Tracing the wound using an appropriate acetate or polythene sheet and a pen is another commonly used method. Photographs may also be taken to provide a visual record of a wound at the time of initial assessment and as it progresses. Whatever method is used, the date that the measurement has been undertaken should be recorded so that it can be compared against later measurements and incorporated into the wound assessment documentation.

DOCUMENTATION

Good documentation is essential in order for all members of the team caring for the patient to obtain a clear picture of the wound and the wound healing journey. Good documentation may also help to identify early signs of complications. Nurses have a legal responsibility to provide good records of all their patient assessments, treatment goals and plan of care as part of their duty of care to patients. The national Nursing and Midwifery Council (NMC) advises that records should include a full account of the assessment and the care planned and provided to patients (NMC, 2007). Many clinical areas have developed

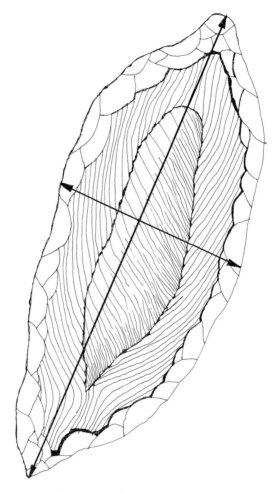

Fig. 5.7 Measuring a wound.

specific charts to use for wound assessment. Fig. 5.8 is an example of a wound assessment chart used for ongoing assessments.

PLANNING
Once a full assessment of both the patient and the wound have been completed, it is possible to plan the most appropriate care. Although the ultimate goal is to heal the wound, it is better to set a series of short-term achievable goals reflecting the stage of healing. As information about the management of different wound types is detailed in Chapter 7, here, planning is described in more general terms with two exemplars that will focus on the wound only. Box 5.1 provides a list of some useful things to remember when selecting a dressing.

Exemplar 1: a pressure ulcer on the heel
- *Assessment* has shown that the patient has a necrotic pressure ulcer on the heel with a hard dry eschar and no exudate. The wound is roughly circular and measures 3 cm in diameter.
- *Treatment aim* is to debride the eschar by encouraging autolysis, or the natural separation of the eschar from the wound bed with the goal of achieving new granulation tissue.
- *Plan of care* needs to take into consideration the difficulty of caring for a wound that is on the heel as well as the need to encourage autolysis by means of 'donating' moisture to the wound eschar to help it to soften and separate. Two types of dressing are very useful in promoting autolysis: hydrogels and hydrocolloids. If the patient is in bed, either of these

Fig. 5.8 Record of wound assessment and dressing plan. Reproduced with kind permission from the University Hospital Birmingham NHS Foundation Trust. © University Hospital Birmingham NHS Foundation Trust.

University Hospital Birmingham NHS Foundation Trust

RECORD OF WOUND ASSESSMENT AND DRESSING PLAN

Complete one form for each of the patient's wounds

Patient ID/ Name / Ward: or Sticker	**Wound site:**
	Type of wound:

Complete this section at initial assessment then weekly or when changes to wound occur

Date and Time				
Grade 1-4 or eschar **(for pressure ulcers only)**				
SIZE (in cms)				
♦ Diameter				
♦ Length				
♦ Depth				
♦ Undermining/fistulas				
♦ Photographed / traced Y / N				
TISSUE TYPE (in %)				
♦ Necrosis/eschar				
♦ Sloughy				
♦ Granulating				
♦ Over granulating				
♦ Other e.g. muscle/bone/adipose				

SURROUNDING SKIN				
♦ Oedema				
♦ Dry/macerated				
♦ Excoriated				
♦ Blanching/nonblanching				
♦ Other e.g. bruising/haematoma				
EXUDATE				
♦ Colour				
♦ Odour				
♦ Quantity e.g. heavy /moderate/ minimum /none				
♦ Type e.g. pus / blood / serous				
INFECTION				
♦ Signs of clinical infection present e.g. Heat/pain/erythema/ pus				
♦ Swab sent?				
♦ Swab results:				
PAIN				
♦ PRN/regular analgesia				
♦ Prior to dressing changes only				
TREATMENT AIMS e.g. manage exudate /deslough/promote granulation/reduce maceration/reduce bacterial load				
COMMENTS				
PRINT NAME				
SIGNATURE				
DESIGNATION				

Referrals to members of the multidisciplinary team

Date and Time	Details:

UHB No: 125

Fig. 5.8 *Continued*

81

Patient ID/ Name / Ward: or Sticker

Mark on the body map position of wound

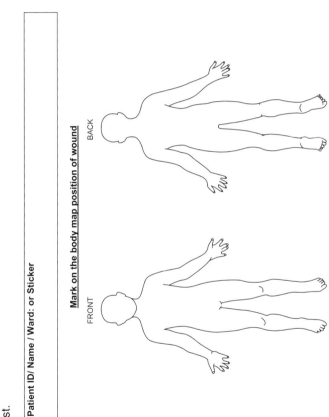

FRONT   BACK

Fig. 5.8 *Continued* Record of wound assessment and dressing plan. Reproduced with kind permission from the University Hospital Birmingham NHS Foundation Trust. © University Hospital Birmingham NHS Foundation Trust.

Dressings Selected - complete at initial assessment and following any changes

Date and Time				
Skin Care/Cleansing Regime				
Primary Dressing				
Secondary Dressing				
Securing Mechanism				
Frequency of Dressing Change				
Print Name				
Signature				
Designation				

Wound Redressed – complete this section following each dressing change

Date and Time		
Comments		
Print Name		
Signature		
Designation		

Date and Time		
Comments		
Print Name:		
Signature		
Designation		

Refer to Wound Dressing Guide and formulary for information on dressing products

TVS 2007   UHB No: 125

Fig. 5.8 *Continued*

83

Box 5.1 Points to consider when selecting a suitable dressing

- Patient comfort, acceptability and expectations
- The level and viscosity of the exudate
- The size and depth of the wound and position of the wound
- The ability of the dressing to achieve optimum moisture balance for the specific wound to promote healing
- Degree of desired mobility is not inhibited by dressing
- The fit of the dressing
- The condition and vulnerability of the surrounding skin (see Chapter 6)
- The suitability of the method of securing the dressing (see Chapter 4)
- Any known allergies to dressing components (see Chapter 6)

Adapted from Cameron, J. (2004) *Nursing Standard* **19**(7): 62–68.

---

types of dressing could be selected, but if the patient is mobile then a hydrocolloid dressing may be more practical as hydrogels may squeeze out from behind the secondary dressing during weight-bearing.

- *Evaluation of progress* should be undertaken on a weekly basis. Once the eschar starts to separate, it may be necessary to review the treatment plan as there may be some offensive exudate requiring more frequent dressing changes. It may be possible to speed the process by using sharp debridement, cutting out the necrotic tissue using scissors or a knife. However, this type of debridement should only be undertaken by a qualified, competent practitioner. Once debridement is complete, further assessment and a new plan of care are required.

Exemplar 2: an abdominal cavity wound

- *Assessment* of this abdominal cavity wound shows that it is full of granulation tissue with little exudate. There are signs of epithelial cells starting to spread across the wound surface. The wound measures 4 cm by 3 cm.
- *Treatment aim* is both to protect the wound and to encourage healing by providing a moist environment at the wound/dressing interface. The goal at this stage is to achieve complete healing.
- *Plan of care* should ensure that a dressing is used that will not stick to the wound and will retain the wound exudate on the wound surface to keep it moist, thus encouraging movement of the epithelial cells. A wide range of dressings could be used, for example: thin foams, films, hydrogels, hydrocolloids and silicone-based dressings. Selection should be based on the position of the wound and the status of the surrounding skin. In this example of an abdominal wound there are no particular problems of dressing retention and the peri-wound skin is normal. Therefore, any of the suggested dressings could be used.
- *Evaluation of progress* will hopefully show complete coverage of the wound with epithelial tissue within a very short time. Once epithelialisation is complete, a simple dry dressing such as a low adherent dressing could be used for a short time to protect the

wound from clothing that might rub on the newly healed wound.

Key points

- Comprehensive wound assessment is key to effective planning.
- Assessment of the patient should be undertaken alongside wound assessment.
- It takes time to develop skills in assessing the wound bed.
- Good documentation is essential to monitor progress of a wound and communication with other members of the multi-professional team.

SUMMARY

This chapter has discussed how to assess a wound and how to use the information to plan appropriate care. Once again, this emphasises the importance of a systematic approach to wound care. The key points provide a reminder of some of the points to consider when planning the care of a wound. There is some cross-referencing to other chapters.

You should now use the knowledge you have gained from reading this chapter and Chapters 3 and 4 to undertake the following exercise.

Exercise 5.1

Case scenario

Mr Alistair Kennedy is a 92-year-old man who has an ulcer on his left lateral malleolus (Fig. 5.9). The ulcer

Continued

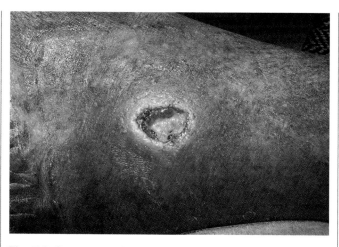

Fig. 5.9 Case scenario: ulcer on the left lateral malleolus.

started as a knock to the ankle and has been present for several months. He was assessed last month in the vascular clinic and offered surgery to improve his arterial blood flow, which he declined. Mr Kennedy is tall and thin and somewhat frail, but is mentally alert and able to answer questions about his health. He walks slowly with a stick and is mainly independent, requiring little help from his wife. The ulcer bed is very sloughy with moderate exudate and measures 2 cm × 1.5 cm in diameter.

Using a systematic approach to help you and using the blank assessment sheet as your guide, consider what your treatment objectives will be for Mr Kennedy and propose a suitable dressing and treatment plan for his sloughy ulcer.

Continued

Step 1: assess the patient, wound and circumstances
When assessing Mr Kennedy you should consider his age, how thin he is, his sleeping position, his lifestyle and his own perceptions of his wound healing. In assessment of the wound itself, you should consider the position of the wound, its depth and the appearance of the wound bed and how this might impact on your dressing choice. Think about how you would document the shape and size of this wound, how you would describe the wound bed and amount and colour of any exudate present, and why this is important.

Step 2: utilise existing information about the patient
You already know that the patient is 92 years old and is mainly independent, with a little support from his wife. His treatment plan should ensure that it does not compromise his lifestyle.

Step 3: explore relevant current best practice
Read through the section on sloughy ulcers in this chapter again and look at the treatment aims. Chapter 4 describes the different dressing types used in the management of different stages of wound healing. You need to consider what type of dressing can be applied to hydrate the wound and promote autolysis (natural breakdown of devitalised tissue such as slough).

Step 4: make a clinical decision
Following the assessment you should have enough information to enable you to make an informed choice as to a suitable dressing for Mr Kennedy's ulcer that will achieve the treatment aims.

Continued

> *Step 5: evaluate progress*
> Think about how you will reassess the ulcer and what you will be looking for to evaluate whether the dressing regimen is effective.

Suggested management

As Mr Kennedy is thin, his assessment should include determining whether he is eating enough, because insufficient nutritional intake can adversely affect healing and the patient might benefit from a food supplement. As part of the assessment Mr Kennedy should be asked what position he likes to sleep in at night and whether he lies on his left side, as this would add pressure over the malleolus where his ulcer is; if possible, he should be encouraged to lie in a different position. Remember that as an older person, Mr Kennedy's wound will heal slowly compared with a younger person's and you should include this fact in your explanation to the patient.

It is also better to set a series of short-term achievable goals reflecting the stages of healing rather than having one overall goal to heal the wound. Good documentation that records wound appearance and dimensions at regular intervals will allow the healthcare team to monitor progress of the wound. The wound exudate should be observed for any changes in quantity or appearance as this may influence the continued suitability of the dressing or frequency of dressing changes. Remember, increased levels of exudate and discolouration may indicate the presence of infection.

Mr Kennedy's dressing should enable him to continue with his daily living activities such as being able to have a shower and being able to wear his shoes so he can walk. A hydrocolloid dressing could be a suitable dressing for this wound as it would hydrate the slough and promote autolysis, encouraging new granulation tissue. A hydrocolloid dressing has a waterproof back and would allow him to continue to shower as normal and as it is not bulky, it would not affect his footwear. Evaluation of Mr Kennedy's ulcer should include evidence that the short-term goals are being met and there are signs of granulation tissue appearing in the wound base. The dressing should continue to be comfortable for him and not interfere unduly with his lifestyle.

CONCLUSION
This exercise has shown you how to use a systematic approach to assess and plan care for a patient with a sloughy wound.

REFERENCES

Cameron, J. (2004) Exudate and care of the peri-wound skin. *Nursing Standard* **19**(7): 62–68.

Cutting, K. & White, R. (2002) Maceration of skin and wound bed, part 1: its nature and cause. *Journal of Wound Care* **11**(7): 275–278.

Nursing and Midwifery Council (2007) *NMC Record Keeping Guidance*. London, Nursing and Midwifery Council.

World Union of Wound Healing Societies (2007) *Principles of Best Practice: Wound Exudate and the Role of Dressings. A Consensus Document.* London, MEP Ltd.

Care of the Peri-Wound Skin

6

INTRODUCTION

This chapter aims to give the reader a fundamental knowledge of the structure and functions of the skin. The problems associated with vulnerable peri-wound skin are discussed with guidance on the assessment process in identifying existing conditions and potential risk factors. Suitable management strategies are described for different types of skin problem. Management of peri-wound skin can be complex and challenging. Nurses have a key role in the decision-making and need a good working knowledge of the different treatment strategies required for the various skin conditions that can present.

THE STRUCTURE OF THE SKIN

The skin is the largest organ in the body, weighing around 3 kg, and when intact forms a protective barrier between the body and the external environment. The skin consists of two layers, the epidermis and the dermis (Fig. 6.1). A layer of subcutaneous fat merges with the deepest layer of the dermis providing thermal insulation and protection from physical forces.

The epidermis

The epidermis is the outermost layer of the skin. It varies in thickness in different parts of the body, being thickest on the soles of the feet and the palms of the hands, and thinnest on the eyelids. The epidermis consists of stratified squamous epithelium divided into five layers:

- *Stratum basale* (basal layer) – in this layer, cells undergo mitosis (i.e. division and reproduction). The cells migrate from the basal layer through each successive layer, until they are shed from the skin surface. The process of cell migration from the stratum basale to outer layers of the stratum corneum takes around 28 days. The basal layer also contains melanocytes, which produce the pigment melanin, and the Langerhans' cells, which are involved in immune function.
- *Stratum spinosum* (prickle cell layer) – the cells initiate protein synthesis required for production of keratin.
- *Stratum granulosum* (granular layer) – the process of keratinisation begins. Cells in this layer have started to degenerate.
- *Stratum lucidum* (clear layer) – the cells are filled with a soft gel-like substance, which is eventually transformed to keratin. This translucent layer is only present where the skin is thickened, on the palms of the hands and soles of the feet.
- *Stratum corneum* (horny layer) – this is the most superficial layer of the epidermis. Cells in the stratum corneum have become filled with keratin. Desmosomes are essential for the maintenance of skin integrity. These are intercellular junctions that hold adjacent keratinocytes together providing extra adhesion and strength (Thibodeau, 1987). The

process of repair and regeneration is continual, as dead surface cells are constantly shed and replaced by cells from the deeper layers. The stratum corneum provides the epidermal barrier to water loss from the skin. The cells of the stratum corneum are embedded in a continuous lipid-enriched cellular matrix. If the skin is continuously exposed to fluid such as wound exudate, incontinence or from excessive washing, loss of lipids occurs and subsequent drying of the epidermis takes place, resulting in impairment of the barrier function of the skin.

Dermal–epidermal junction

The area of contact between the basal layer of the epidermis and dermis is called the basement membrane and is made largely from collagens. A series of undulated ridges projecting down from the epidermis and peaks projecting up from the dermis give strength to the skin and prevent separation of the epidermis and dermis (Bale *et al.*, 2006). Blistering can occur if the epidermis becomes separated from the dermis due to excessive shear forces at the epidermis–dermis interface (Cosker *et al.*, 2005).

The dermis

The dermis is thicker than the epidermis and is composed of collagen, reticulum and elastin fibres, which form a framework to support the nerve endings, blood vessels, lymphatic capillaries, sweat glands, sebaceous glands and hair follicles. The sweat glands (eccrine, apocrine) pass through the epidermis and open on the skin surface through the pores. Water, salts and toxins are excreted through the sweat glands. The sebaceous

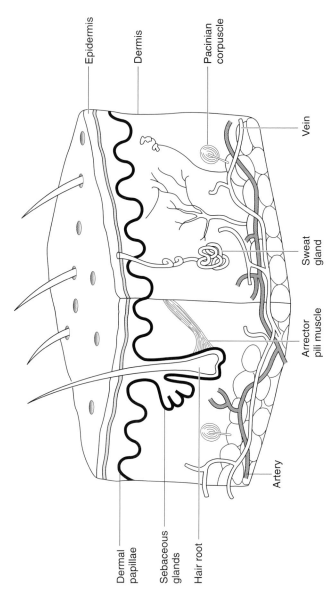

Fig. 6.1 Cross-section of the skin.

Epidermis

Dermis

Pacinian corpuscle

Vein

Sweat gland

Arrector pili muscle

Artery

Dermal papillae

Sebaceous glands

Hair root

glands open into a hair follicle and secrete sebum. The deepest layer of the dermis merges into the subcutaneous tissue or hypodermis, which provides thermal insulation (Thibodeau, 1987). The hypodermis contains both connective tissue and adipose tissue and helps to anchor the skin to muscle and bone. See Fig. 6.1 for a diagrammatic illustration of the cross-section of the skin.

FUNCTIONS OF THE SKIN
Protection
The skin forms a protective covering for the body. The natural acid pH of the skin's surface inhibits bacterial production and protects the body from bacterial invasion. Melanocytes synthesise melanin resulting in darkening of the skin. The pigment protects the body from ultra-violet radiation damage (Butcher & White, 2005). The sensory receptors in the dermis warn the body of pain, temperature changes, pressure and touch. Different types of sensory receptor respond to the various forms of external stimuli. A reflex action occurs in response to a sensory stimulus as part of the body's ability to protect itself from damage.

Temperature regulation
In normal healthy humans the body temperature is maintained at around 37 °C. The skin plays a major role in maintaining this constant level of body temperature. Heat regulation is controlled by vasodilation for cooling and vasoconstriction for warming.

Vasodilation occurs when the body becomes too warm. Loss of heat is under the control of the autonomic nervous system. During increased heat production, as a result of exercise or from external temperature, blood vessels become dilated, allowing more blood to reach the surface of the skin. This produces a reddening of the skin (in the face and sometimes in other parts of the body as well). Sweating occurs simultaneously and evaporation of perspiration from the skin has a cooling effect on the body.

Vasoconstriction occurs when the body becomes too cold. Blood vessels in the skin contract as a result of the activity of the vasoconstrictor nerves. Vasoconstriction of blood vessels redirects blood and therefore heat from the extremities to the internal organs to ensure they are kept warm. As a result the skin becomes pale in appearance. Rapid cooling of the body surface causes shivering and the arrector pili muscles, attached to hair follicles, contract causing body hair to stand on end. The reflex action of shivering, causing rapid and repeated muscle contractions, works to increase heat and raise body temperature. Putting warm clothing or other coverings such as blankets on a person who is cold assists in preventing the process of heat loss.

Sensation

Normal skin is sensitive to pain, touch, temperature and pressure, through its network of nerve endings or receptors. When stimulated these receptors transmit impulses or signals to the cerebral cortex where they are interpreted (Bale *et al.*, 2006). Patients in whom the skin barrier function has become impaired may experience sensations of stinging, itching or burning due to increased sensory stimulus to the skin (Cameron, 2006).

FACTORS INFLUENCING PERI-WOUND SKIN BREAKDOWN

- The ageing process adversely affects the skin, which tends to be dry and vulnerable and particularly at risk of breakdown (Davies, 1992).
- Skin dryness may cause generalised itching and a reduction in barrier function.
- Peri-wound skin has been found to have a compromised barrier function compared to normal skin (Bishop *et al.*, 2003).
- The use of inappropriate wound dressings can lead to skin trauma (Cameron, 2006).
- Leakage of excessive exudate will damage vulnerable peri-wound skin, leading to skin breakdown and increased serous fluid loss, adversely influencing the healing outcome (Cameron, 2004).

SKIN ASSESSMENT

The assessment should include a comprehensive assessment of the patient's skin, together with a detailed clinical history. When taking the clinical history it is important to establish and document the following:

- Any known skin problems and conditions, such as eczema.
- Medication and the effect it may have had on the skin, e.g. long-term steroids may have left the skin thin and vulnerable.
- Degree of mobility. Immobility can leave patients vulnerable to skin damage from undue pressure.
- Position of patient during the day and at night (some patients sit in a chair all night).

- Current and past use of dressings and emollients that have caused adverse effects on the skin.
- Known allergies to dressings and skin care products (some patients may have already been patch tested).
- Age of patient. Ageing can affect the resilience of the skin tissues.

Examining the patient's skin

The aim of the skin examination is to identify existing skin problems and potential risk factors. Any existing conditions and loss of skin integrity should be documented. Newton and Cameron (2003) recommend a five-step approach (*colour, texture, temperature, sensation, integrity*) in their guidelines for skin assessment and the potential causes of damage in the peri-wound area.

Colour

- *Examination*: check the skin for changes to normal skin tone such as erythema, bluish tones, brown staining and bruising.
- *Possible causes*: erythema (redness) may be an indication of inflammation or unrelieved pressure. Brown staining on the skin of the lower leg is an indication of venous disease.
- *Assessing dark skin*: normal skin colour varies from person to person and early skin changes are difficult to see in very dark skin. The assessment is based on changes in skin temperature and tissue consistency (Dealey & Lindholm, 2006).

Texture

- *Examination*: check if the skin is dry and inelastic. Is there any scaling or crusting? Are there any moist or soggy areas, or is the skin oedematous?
- *Possible causes*: dry and inelastic skin occurs in older patients and may be associated with muscle wastage, making the skin vulnerable to skin tears. Moist, erythematous and shiny skin indicates an acute condition, which could be due to exudate damage or may be contact dermatitis. Scaling and crusting indicate an eczematous condition. Soggy white skin indicates prolonged exposure to wound fluid. Oedematous skin may be due to inflammation, limb dependency, venous insufficiency, cardiac disease and malnutrition.

Temperature

- *Examination*: normal skin temperature should feel warm to the touch. If the patient's skin feels hot, check their temperature and ask if they feel generally unwell. If the skin feels hot in a localised area check the colour, texture and sensation to help in the diagnosis.
- *Possible causes*: erythema, heat, pain and swelling indicate inflammation/infection. Cold skin with pallor and/or bluish tones indicate poor vascularisation in the area.

Sensation

- *Symptoms*: the many different skin conditions cause varying sensations and patients may complain that their skin feels sore or painful or is burning, itching or stinging or that they have tingling or loss of feeling.

- *Possible causes*: itching may be due to dryness, contact dermatitis or varicose eczema. Burning and stinging plus redness and moisture may be due to erythematous maceration, where wound exudate has become trapped against the skin. Pain may be due to an inappropriate dressing adhering to the wound. Heat, erythema and swelling together with the sensation of pain indicate the presence of infection/inflammation in the tissues.

Integrity

- *Examination*: check the peri-wound area for any skin breaks, epidermal stripping, skin tears or blisters.
- *Possible causes*: this type of trauma can be caused by inappropriate use of dressings and bandages on vulnerable skin or even poor manual handling. It is advisable to avoid using adhesive dressings and tapes on fragile oedematous tissue to prevent skin trauma. Older patients with frail skin are particularly vulnerable to this type of skin damage.

MANAGEMENT OF THE PERI-WOUND SKIN

The aim of management is to keep the peri-wound skin clean, dry and protected from trauma.

How excessive wound exudate damages skin

Exudate from chronic wounds appears to have a damaging effect on normal wound healing due to raised levels of tissue destructive enzymes (Trengove *et al.*, 1999, Drinkwater *et al.*, 2002). The role of exudate and how it affects wound healing is discussed in detail in Chapter 1. Prolonged exposure to chronic wound exudate on previously healthy skin will result in maceration and may facilitate further loss of epithelium. The appearance of maceration varies according to the amount of local inflammation present. 'White maceration' occurs when there is maceration but little inflammation. The peri-wound skin appears white, hard and swollen. Application of a suitable skin protectant to the peri-wound area can prevent skin damage from wound exudate and reduce the risk of further loss of epithelium. Maceration damage may also result in the peri-wound skin being red, inflamed, moist or weeping. This is termed 'erythematous maceration' as opposed to white maceration (Newton & Cameron, 2004).

The initial treatment of erythematous maceration is different from that of white maceration. A topical steroid preparation may be prescribed, for a few days only, to reduce any local inflammation present. The topical steroid relieves the symptoms of stinging and soreness within 24 hours and after 2–3 days treatment can continue with regular use of a skin protectant. Zinc paste and a skin protectant that leaves a protective film on the surface have both been shown to be effective barrier preparations, when used around leg ulcers (Cameron *et al.*, 2005). The addition of a 50% white soft paraffin/50% liquid paraffin mixture (50/50) is required when applying zinc paste on very moist skin and also for removal. A barrier film is widely used as a barrier preparation on peri-ulcer skin and is available as an impregnated sponge on a stick or in a spray.

Varicose eczema

A complicating factor in the management of venous leg ulcers is the presence of eczema on the skin of the lower leg. Care must be taken when applying any dressings and bandages to the skin of a patient with weeping eczema to prevent adhesion to the peri-wound skin. If there is adhesion to the skin the limb should be soaked in warm water prior to removal of the dressings and bandages to avoid unnecessary pain and trauma to the patient. Adhesive dressings are best avoided on eczematous skin. Varicose eczema is managed with compression therapy to address the underlying venous dysfunction and, if severe, a topical steroid ointment may be prescribed. Topical steroids have an anti-inflammatory effect and decrease cell division in the epidermis.

Topical steroids are divided into four groups according to their potency:

• Mildly potent
• Moderately potent
• Potent
• Very potent

The potency of the topical steroid required depends on the severity of the eczema. Topical steroids should be applied thinly to the affected area in a downward stroke and not rubbed into the skin. Topical steroids should be used for a few days only and then treatment continued with a simple emollient such as '50/50' (50% white soft paraffin / 50% liquid paraffin).

Allergic contact dermatitis

Allergic contact dermatitis is caused by direct contact with external substances and is particularly common in patients with venous leg ulcers. An allergen sensitises through skin contact. On renewed contact with the allergen sensitised lymphocytes are reactivated via the skin and circulation (Sibbald & Cameron, 2001). The allergic response is seen clinically as inflamed skin, characterised by erythema, weeping and scaling in the area of direct contact with the responsible agent (Fig. 6.2) (Scheper *et al.*, 1992). Itchy skin is often a predominant symptom of allergic contact dermatitis. Research studies have shown that it is possible for a patient with a venous leg ulcer to become allergic to any part of their topical treatment including dressings, emollients, creams, bandages and latex gloves

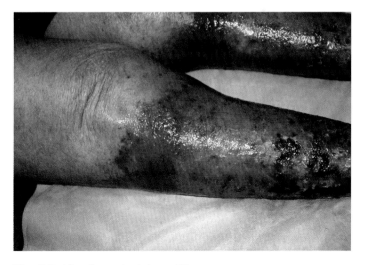

Fig. 6.2 Allergic contact dermatitis.

worn by the carer (Gooptu & Powell, 1999; Tavadia *et al.*, 2003; Machet *et al.*, 2004). If an allergic contact dermatitis is suspected the patient should be referred to a dermatologist for patch testing so the causal agent can be identified and subsequently avoided in future management (Cameron, 2006).

Dry scaly skin

Dry skin tends to be itchy and scratching increases the risk of skin breakdown. Dry skin is managed with emollients to prevent water loss and lubricate the skin. Application of an emollient to affected areas will leave a layer of oil on the skin and thus reduce transepidermal water loss. Emollients may be ointments or creams. Ointments are greasy preparations mainly with a paraffin base and have little or no water. They are more occlusive than creams and maintain hydration longer. Patients with chronic venous insufficiency who have thick dry skin scale (hyperkeratosis) on their lower legs should have their legs immersed in warm water for 10–20 minutes to soften the scale before applying an emollient. A simple emollient, such as '50/50', should be applied regularly, to loosen the scale and keep the skin hydrated (Cameron, 1998). Treatment needs to be frequent and long term as the skin scale can quickly build up again. Creams are an emulsion of oil in water or water in oil, in semi-solid form. When applied to the skin most evaporates due to the high water content and a thin film of oil is left on the skin surface. Creams are often more acceptable to patients and carers as they are less greasy than ointments and easily absorbed into the skin. However, creams contain preservatives and other additives and are therefore best avoided on the skin around venous leg ulcers.

Skin stripping

Skin damage to previously healthy peri-wound skin can occur from repeated application and removal of adhesive dressings and tapes, eliciting changes to the barrier function and superficial hydration of the skin (Dykes *et al.*, 2001; Zillmer *et al.*, 2006). This may lead to an inflammatory skin reaction in some patients. The clinical appearance is similar to an allergic reaction. A barrier preparation that leaves a protective film on the skin surface (as described above) may be applied under adhesive dressings to aid adhesion and prevent trauma on removal.

Key points

- The skin is the largest organ in the body and repairs and regenerates itself continually.
- The process of cell migration from the stratum basale to outer layers of the stratum corneum takes around 28 days.
- The stratum corneum provides the epidermal barrier to water loss from the skin.
- Factors that influence skin breakdown include ageing skin, position and mobility, mechanical and chemical trauma.
- All patients should have a comprehensive assessment of their skin to identify existing skin problems and potential risk factors.
- The aim of management is to keep the peri-wound skin clean, dry and protected from trauma.

Continued

- The ageing process leaves skin vulnerable and more susceptible to breakdown.
- Dry skin is managed with emollients.
- Skin that is exposed to moisture should be protected with a suitable barrier preparation.
- If an allergy is suspected the patient should be referred to a dermatologist.

SUMMARY

This chapter has focused on giving you a basic understanding of the structure and functions of the skin together with how to assess the skin and manage some of the problems associated with vulnerable peri-wound skin. You should now use the knowledge you have gained from reading this chapter to undertake the following exercise.

Exercise 6.1

Case scenario

Mr Rogers has attended the leg ulcer clinic today. He is 78 years old and has a long-standing venous leg ulcer, which has been healing well. His wife Jean is disabled and he is the main carer. Jean has been waking frequently in the night over the past week due to a persistent cough following a bad cold and he has been getting up to help her. Mr Rogers is keeping well in himself although he does get tired. He is complaining today that his skin around the ulcer feels very sore with a stinging sensation. After removing the bandage and dressings you

Continued

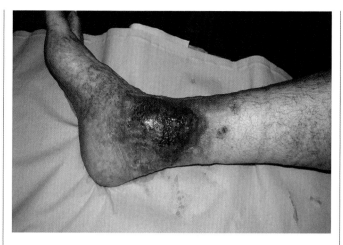

Fig. 6.3 Case scenario: erythematous maceration.

examine the wound and skin. The skin is very red and moist (see Fig. 6.3).

How will you determine what treatment to start? Using a systematic approach, think about how you will go about this.

Step 1: assess the patient, wound and circumstances

In your assessment you should consider the colour and texture of the skin. Look at the assessment guidelines given in this chapter and determine possible causes for the colour and texture of the peri-wound skin.

Step 2: utilise existing information about the patient

Consider what you already know and what you might want to ask the patient to help in your diagnosis.

Continued

Step 3: explore relevant current best practice
What are the recommendations for protecting the skin around a venous leg ulcer? Is there research to support this?

Step 4: make a clinical decision
When you have found the answers to the above questions you should be able to consider what may have caused the skin problem and how you could plan Mr Rogers' care.

Step 5: evaluate progress
Think about when you would want to see Mr Rogers again to evaluate whether the treatment has been successful.

Suggested management

The skin around Mr Rogers' leg ulcer is very red and moist. Possible causes of this could be due to trapped exudate causing erythematous maceration or it may be an allergy or due to infection. You need to establish whether he has any pain and whether there is any odour present, as this may indicate infection. The information you have already is that his ulcer has been healing well and that he has been getting little rest recently because his wife has been unwell. If his skin was very itchy, that would indicate a possible contact dermatitis. Mr Rogers has stated that his skin feels sore and stinging, which indicates possible erythematous maceration, caused by excessive wound exudate coming into contact with the skin. He has been on his feet a lot more than usual caring for his wife and this may have caused an increase in wound exudate production.

You should also establish whether Mr Rogers has been able to attend all his appointments for dressing changes or if the dressing has been in place for longer than usual. Treatment of erythematous maceration is by first reducing the local inflammation with a topical steroid ointment, which would require a prescription, then applying a skin protectant. Research has shown that allergic reactions are particularly common in patients who have venous leg ulcers and a simple skin protectant such as zinc paste or a skin protectant that leaves a protective film on the skin surface is recommended. Mr Rogers should be told that the stinging and itching should stop in 24 hours. Another appointment should be made for him in 3 days' time to check his skin and apply the skin protectant.

CONCLUSION

This exercise has shown you how to work through the decision-making process in a systematic way to enable you to reach an informed decision about what may be causing Mr Rogers' skin problem and how his care can be planned and managed.

REFERENCES

Bale, S., Cameron, J. & Meaume, S. (2006) Skin care. In: Romanelli, M. (ed.) *Science and Practice of Pressure Ulcer Management.* London, Springer-Verlag.

Bishop, S.M., Walker, M., Rogers, A.A. & Chen, W.Y.J. (2003) Importance of moisture balance at the wound-dressing interface. *Journal of Wound Care* **12**(4): 125–128.

Butcher, M. & White, R. (2005) The structure and functions of the skin. In: White, R. (ed.) *Skin Care in Wound Management: Assessment, Prevention, Treatment.* Aberdeen, Wounds UK Ltd.

Cameron, J. (1998) Skin care for patients with chronic leg ulcers. *Journal of Wound Care* **7**(9): 459–462.

Cameron, J. (2004) Exudate and care of the peri-wound skin. *Nursing Standard* **19**(7): 62–68.

Cameron, J. (2006) Allergic reactions to treatment. In: White, R. & Harding, K. (eds) *Trauma and Pain in Wound Care.* Aberdeen, Wounds UK Ltd.

Cameron, J., Hofman, D., Wilson, J. & Cherry, G. (2005) Comparison of two peri-wound skin protectants in venous leg ulcers; a randomised controlled trial. *Journal of Wound Care* **14**(5): 233–236.

Cosker, T., Elsayed, S., Gupta, S. *et al.* (2005) Choice of dressing has a major impact on blistering and healing outcomes in orthopaedic patients. *Journal of Wound Care* **14**(1): 27–30.

Davies, I. (1992) The mechanisms of ageing. In: Graham-Brown, R.A.C. & Monk, B.E. (eds) *Skin Disorders in the Elderly.* Oxford, Blackwell Scientific Publications.

Dealey, C. & Lindholm, C. (2006) Pressure ulcer classification. In: Romaelli, M. (ed.) *Science and Practice of Pressure Ulcer Management.* London, Springer-Verlag.

Drinkwater, S.L., Smith, A., Sawyer, B.M. & Barnard, K.G. (2002) Effect of venous ulcer exudates on angiogenesis in vitro. *British Journal of Surgery* **89**(6): 709–713.

Dykes, P., Heggle, R. & Hill, S.A. (2001) Effects of adhesive dressings on the stratum corneum. *Journal of Wound Care* **10**(2): 7–10.

Gooptu, C. & Powell, S.M. (1999) The problems of rubber hypersensitivity (types I and IV) in chronic leg and stasis eczema patients. *Contact Dermatitis* **41**: 89–93.

Machet, L., Couhe, C., Perrinaud, A., Hoarau, C., Lorette, G. & Vaillant, L. (2004) A high prevalence of sensitization still persists in leg ulcer patients: a retrospective series of 106 patients tested between 2001 and 2002 and a meta-analysis of 1975–2003 data. *British Journal of Dermatology* **150**(5): 929–935.

Newton, H. & Cameron, J. (2004) *Skin Care in Wound Management*. A clinical education in wound management booklet. Holsworthy, Medical Communications UK Ltd.

Scheper, R.J. & von Blomberg, M. (1992) Cellular mechanisms in allergic contact dermatitis. In: Rycroft, R.G.J., Menné, T., Frosch, P.J. & Benezra, C. (eds) *Textbook of Contact Dermatitis*. Berlin, Springer-Verlag.

Sibbald, R.G. & Cameron, J. (2001) Dermatological aspects of wound care. In: Krasner, D.L., Rodeheaver, G.T. & Sibbald, R.G. (eds) *Chronic Wound Care: A Clinical Source Book for Healthcare Professionals, Third Edition*. Wayne, PA, HMP Communications.

Tavadia, S., Bianchi, J., Dawe, R.S., McEvoy, M., Wiggins, E., Hamill, E., Urcelay, M., Strong, A.M. & Douglas, W.S. (2003) Allergic contact dermatitis in venous leg ulcer patients. *Contact Dermatitis* **48**: 261–265.

Thibodeau, G.A. (1987) The skin and its appendages. In: Thibodeau, G.A. (ed.) *Anatomy and Physiology*. St Louis, MO, Times Mirror/ Mosby College Publishing.

Trengove, N.J., Stacey, M.C., MacAuley, S., Bennett, N., Gibson, J., Burslem, F., Murphy, G & Schultz, G. (1999) Analysis of the acute and chronic wound environments: the role of proteases and their inhibitors. *Wound Repair and Regeneration* **7**: 42–52.

Zillmer, R., Agren, M.S., Gottrup, F. & Kalsmark, T. (2006) Biophysical effects of repetitive removal of adhesive dressings on peri-ulcer skin. *Journal of Wound Care* **15**(5): 187–191.

Management of Wounds

INTRODUCTION

This chapter focuses on the management of specific types of wounds. It needs to be read in conjunction with Chapter 3, which discusses the factors that can affect healing, and Chapter 4, which provides a framework for the general principles of wound management. Chapter 2 provides information about the epidemiology of the wounds which are discussed here.

This chapter is divided into two sections covering acute and chronic wounds. Only the most frequently occurring types of wound are discussed here; detailed information about all types of wounds can be found in Dealey (2005).

ACUTE WOUNDS

Surgical wounds

Generally, surgical wounds will heal without problem and only a minority will develop complications. The overarching aim when caring for patients with surgical wounds is detection of early signs of complications.

Methods of closure

Once an operative procedure is completed, the layers of different tissues that have been cut open have to be repaired. In most cases, the layers of tissue are sutured and the skin edges brought together and held in approximation by sutures, clips, staples or tape depending on the position of the wound and the preference of the surgeon. Sutures, sometimes called stitches, can be made from a variety of materials such as nylon and silk, and they are removed between 7 and 14 days after surgery, depending on the position of the wound. Clips and staples are made of metal and require special applicators for applying and removing them. They are generally removed between 5 and 7 days after surgery. There are also specially made tapes for holding skin edges together, which are narrow and come cut to length. The tapes may be left in place for 7–14 days.

For some operations it is not appropriate to close the skin in this way, usually because there is a high risk of infection or the need to allow drainage from the wound. In these instances the inner layers of tissue are closed and the outer layers left open to heal from the base of the wound. This is called healing by secondary intention, whereas healing with the skin edges closed is called healing by primary intention. In order to prevent the wound closing too quickly, the cavity is filled with a dressing material such as alginate.

Dressings

Wounds healing by primary intention will epithelialise within 48 hours, which seals the wound. Mangram *et al.* (1999) state that there is no good evidence to suggest that a dressing is required after this time. However, dressings provide protection for the wound against rubbing by clothing and improve patient comfort (Briggs, 1996). Birchall and Taylor (2003) suggest that an appropriate dressing for a surgical wound should be absorbent, low adherent and semi-permeable. In addition, Watret and White (2001) proposed that the dressing should be conformable, easy to use and cost-effective. Probably the commonest type of dressing used is an island dressing, which meets all the above criteria. Other types of dressing in regular use are films, thin hydrocolloids and foams. Film dressings have the advantage of being able to view the wound without having to remove the dressing, but, unless they specifically incorporate an absorbent pad, they have no absorbency.

Complications

A number of complications can occur, the commonest of which are haemorrhage, infection or breakdown of the suture line, known as dehiscence. Haemorrhage can occur during the operation or in the post-operative period. It may be due to uncontrolled bleeding during the operation, a slipped suture around a blood vessel or, if it occurs late in the post-operative period, infection. The bleeding needs to be controlled and may require further surgery to do so. If there is excessive bleeding, the patient may require a blood transfusion.

Infection can occur in around 10% of surgical wounds (Emmerson *et al.*, 1996). Although there may be several different factors involved, poor surgical technique is the commonest cause of infection (Dealey, 2005). Some types of surgery have a higher risk of infection than others. For example, surgery to repair a perforated appendix carries a much higher risk of infection than varicose vein surgery. When there is a known risk of infection, patients are usually given antibiotic prophylaxis.

Wound dehiscence may occur along part or all of a suture line (Fig. 7.1). There are a variety of reasons for the dehiscence, such as infection, poor suturing technique or the sutures being removed too soon. Generally, if dehiscence occurs along part of a suture line it is left open to heal by granulation. These wounds can be quite sloughy with a moderate to heavy amount of exudate, depending on the size and depth of the wound. Appropriate dressings may be alginates or hydrofibre dressings for deep wounds with heavy

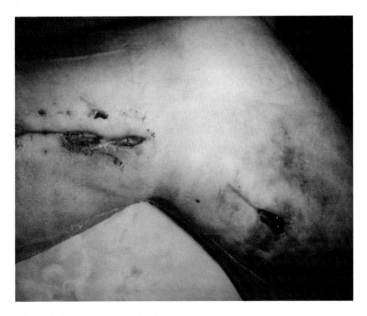

Fig. 7.1 Dehiscent surgical wounds.

exudate or an amorphous hydrogel for shallower wounds.

Monitoring progress

Nurses have a responsibility to monitor surgical wounds closely for any indication of complications. Ideally, this should be undertaken at least 4 hourly for the first 12 hours after surgery and then daily until the skin closures are removed. As patients are often discharged after a few days this is not always possible. Patients should be given written and verbal advice on the possible indicators of complications and the actions to be taken should they occur.

Patient management

Most patients find the experience of having an operation quite daunting. Many may have never been in hospital before. An important aspect of nursing care is to alleviate anxiety by ensuring that patients are given clear information about the whole process so that they know what to expect. Every patient is entitled to effective post-operative pain management and patients require assessment and appropriate analgesia. Chapter 8 gives more information about pain management.

Some patients will require specific care because of pre-existing conditions such as diabetes. Others will require following a regimen of care specific to their type of surgery. For example, patients undergoing orthopaedic surgery may have to limit their range of movement, whereas patients undergoing gastrointestinal surgery will not be able to return to a normal diet immediately after their operation.

Traumatic wounds

Major trauma or complex injury is beyond the remit of this book. The commonest minor traumatic injuries are cuts, abrasions and lacerations and these will be discussed here. There are some basic principles of overall patient assessment that need to be followed when assessing any patient with a traumatic injury (Small, 2000).

Patient history

Find out when and how the injury occurred, taking into account that some injuries may not be accidental. Accident and emergency departments have policies for dealing with suspected non-accidental injuries, particularly in children and older people.

- Make a record of any first-aid treatment that has already been applied to the wound.
- Determine the patient's tetanus immunisation status and whether booster immunisation is required.
- Determine if the patient has any allergies, especially to wound care items such as adhesive tapes.
- Determine the patient's social circumstances, whether the patient lives alone and if assistance is available if required.
- If the wound is likely to be disfiguring, then there may be psychological issues to address, either immediately or at a later stage.
- Assessment of the level of pain experienced by the patient is important as it may be necessary to provide analgesia before any treatment can commence. Pain and its management is dealt with in more detail in Chapter 8.

Wound assessment

- Chapter 5 provides detailed information on general wound assessment and should be read in conjunction with the specific information included here.
- Ensure that the full extent of any traumatic wound is clearly seen and assess the wound to estimate the amount of bleeding that has occurred; it should be borne in mind that head wounds bleed heavily.
- Any tissue loss should be identified – this involves assessing whether any of the skin's epidermis has retracted away from the dermis, or if there is complete loss of the epidermis or deeper layers of tissue.
- Determine if there is any loss of function of the affected part or loss of sensation. For example, if a patient has a deep cut to a finger, check if he or she can move and bend it.
- When a hand is injured, check if it is the dominant hand or not.
- Although medical assessment and intervention may be required in many situations, skilled nurses may manage some of the minor injuries.

Wound cleansing

Before applying any form of treatment, it is essential to ensure that the wound has been thoroughly cleaned to remove any foreign bodies, such as grit or embedded clothing, from the wound. By their very nature, traumatic wounds are likely to be heavily contaminated with bacteria and so at great risk of infection, especially if the injury occurred some hours previously. Cleansing is best achieved by using either normal saline or tap water.

Management of cuts

- Cuts are caused by a sharp instrument and there is no tissue loss. The aims of treatment are to control any bleeding and to hold the skin edges together to allow healing. Depending on the position and depth of the cut, it can be managed in a variety of ways, such as sutures, adhesive strips or tissue adhesives.
- Sutures should be used on cuts over joints or on cuts on the hand (Dealey, 2005). Their application requires considerable skill so that there is no scarring, especially if used to manage cuts on the face.
- Adhesive strips can be useful if the patient has fragile skin which might tear if sutures are applied. However, they should not be used over joints as they are likely to pull away from the skin if stretched.
- Tissue adhesives (or glues) can be very useful, especially for treating children as they can be applied quickly and painlessly (Farion *et al.*, 2004). They can be very useful in treating cuts on the head as only a very small area of hair needs to be shaved off compared with the amount needing to be shaved off to apply sutures.

Management of abrasions

Abrasions are superficial injuries where the surface of the skin has rubbed against a hard surface and there is little or no bleeding. It is the type of injury that can occur as a result of falling onto gravel or similar surfaces. Abrasions often have foreign bodies such as grit embedded in them and if they are not completely removed they can cause long-term scarring, sometimes called tattooing (Small, 2000). Abrasions often

119

feel very sore and may benefit from being covered with a film dressing or thin hydrocolloid or adhesive foam dressing.

Management of pre-tibial lacerations

A laceration is a tear in the skin caused by a blunt instrument or force and has a jagged edge. Pre-tibial lacerations are the commonest type of skin laceration (see Chapter 2) and older people are particularly vulnerable as their skin is thinner and less elastic (Ratcliff & Fletcher, 2007). Severe lacerations, where there is a large haematoma and possibly necrosis of the skin flap or where there is a major degloving injury, require surgery. Simple lacerations, even with a small haematoma or skin-edge necrosis, can be managed conservatively. Any haematoma should be evacuated and any necrosis trimmed, after which the skin edges can be brought together and adhesive strips applied as shown in Fig. 7.2. Pre-tibial lacerations should have a supportive bandage applied from toe to knee.

Aftercare

Some patients may require assistance at home, especially for wounds affecting the hand, as simple, everyday tasks may be difficult to carry out. If this is the case they should be encouraged to seek help from family or friends. Patients should also be encouraged to mobilise as much as possible. If the injury affects a limb or digit, it is helpful to elevate the affected part when resting in order to reduce oedema. Simple analgesia may be required for a few days if the wound is sore.

The wound needs to be reviewed by a healthcare professional at day 7 and possibly day 14 in a hospital

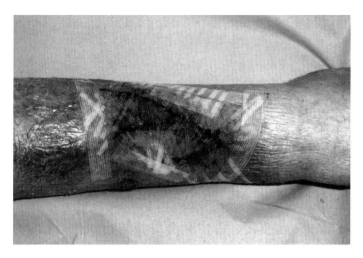

Fig. 7.2 Adhesive tapes applied to a pre-tibial laceration.

clinic or GP surgery (Dunkin *et al.*, 2003). The majority of wounds will heal without complication, but there is a risk of infection in these wounds. Patients should be advised to seek medical assistance if the wound becomes swollen and inflamed or the level of pain suddenly increases.

Burns

Burns are caused by heat, chemicals, electricity, sunlight or radiation. Scalds may be caused by contact with hot fluids, steam or flammable liquids or gases. The severity of the burn is measured in terms of the depth of skin damage and the spread of the damage. Skin depth is measured in terms of:

- Superficial: when only the epithelial layer of skin is damaged. The skin looks red and may be swollen and feels very sore. This is commonly seen in sun burn.
- Partial thickness: the damage penetrates through the epidermis and into the dermis. The skin will be red and swollen with blisters and there may be some weeping from the surface. The area will be painful.
- Deep: both the epidermis and dermis are damaged. The skin is dry and leathery in appearance. There is usually little or no pain because the nerve endings have been destroyed.

The spread of the burn injury is measured in terms of the percentage of the body that is affected and is measured using the 'rule of nines' (Fig. 7.3) (Wallace, 1951). Thus, if a small child knocked over a cup of hot tea, and it spilled over his arm and chest this would total 27% of the total body surface area (TBSA) (9% for the arm and 18% for the chest). An extensive burn can be defined as a burn that covers more than 15% of an adult's body or 10% of the body of a child or older adult, and requires care in a specialist burns unit (Alsbjörn *et al.*, 2007); their management is beyond the remit of this book. A group of European burn specialists recommend a number of other circumstances (see Table 7.1) when patients should be referred to a specialist burns unit. They have also made recommendations on the management of partial thickness burns (Alsbjörn *et al.*, 2007). Management is considered in terms of first aid, initial assessment, the management of superficial and partial thickness burns and after care.

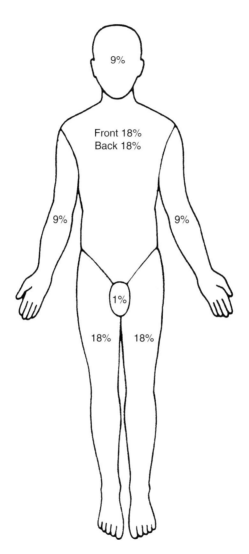

Fig. 7.3 Rule of nines.

Table 7.1 When patients with burn injuries should be referred to a specialist burn unit.

Time of referral	Type of burn
Initial	All full thickness burns
	>15% TBSA in adults
	>10% TBSA in children and older people
	Burns to face, neck, axilla, hands, genitalia, popliteal region, feet
	Circumferential burns
	Electrical or chemical burns
	Non-accidental burns
	Burns associated with inhalational injury, trauma or disease
Late	Burns not healed in 10–14 days
	Late onset of fever, pain, malaise, redness, odour, increased exudate
Very late	Hypertrophic scarring or contractures

Based on Alsbjörn *et al.* (2007).
TBSA, total body surface area.

First aid for burns

The basic first-aid treatment for a burn is the same, regardless of the severity of the injury. The guidance below is provided by St John's Ambulance (SJA, 2007).

- The area affected needs to be cooled straight away to prevent the burned area extending. This is best achieved by placing the affected part under cold running water for at least 10 minutes.
- Wearing disposable gloves, remove jewellery, watch or clothing from the affected area, unless it is stuck to the skin.

- The burn should be covered with cling film, a plastic bag or a non-fluffy material. Do not use any form of adhesives on the skin.
- The urgency with which medical assistance is sought depends on the severity of the burn injury. If the individual has a major or extensive burn, help is required immediately.
- Creams or ointments should not be applied in the first instance.
- Blisters should not be broken.

Assessment

Assessment must be undertaken to determine the depth and extent of the injury, recognising that the depth of injury is unlikely to be uniform across the extent of a large burn. As burn injuries can be very painful, a pain assessment should also be undertaken and appropriate analgesia provided as soon as possible. The patient's tetanus status should be checked and vaccination given if necessary. Having a burn or scald can be very frightening, especially for children, and levels of anxiety should be determined and reassurance given. Once it is determined that it is not necessary to refer the patient to a burns unit, a plan of action can be developed.

Managing superficial burns

There is little evidence to support the management of superficial burns, but in general the treatment consists of application of moisturising cream liberally to the affected area (Reg & Johnson, 2002; Prodigy Guidance, 2004). These creams have a soothing effect and often feel cool to the overheated skin. Superficial burns gen-erally heal in a few days, although the epidermis may peel off after 1–2 days.

Managing partial thickness burns

The burn is likely to be clean if it had been possible to place the affected area under a cold running tap in the early stages. Any loose skin should be removed prior to applying a dressing. Some partial thickness burns may form blisters and there is a lack of agreement about how they may best be managed (Sargent, 2006). Alsbjörn *et al.* (2007) recommend that blisters less than 2% TBSA should be punctured and drained whereas larger blisters should be removed. Either procedure should only be undertaken by a competent, qualified nurse or doctor. The burn injury should be covered with a dressing which will help to keep the wound surface moist while absorbing any excess exudate. Suitable dressings include alginates, foams, hydrocol-loids, and silicone dressings. Specific dressing selection depends on the location of the burn and the ability of the dressing to conform to the contours of the skin (see also Chapter 5). Ideally, the selected dressing should not require frequent changing, as dressing removal can be painful for the patient. Burn wounds should be monitored for any indications of infection and failure to heal within 10–14 days necessitates referral to a burns unit.

Aftercare

Superficial and partial thickness burns should heal without scarring. However, it is important to teach patients to moisturise the healed burn regularly using lotions or creams. If the burn site becomes very itchy despite the application of moisturisers, medical advice should be sought as oral medication may be required (Alsbjörn *et al.*, 2007). Patients must also be advised to protect themselves from the sun by avoiding exposure as much as possible and, when it is not possible, to apply sunscreen with a sun protection factor (SPF) of at least 25 (Alsbjörn *et al.*, 2007).

Abnormal scarring may occasionally occur in the form of hypertrophic scars where the scar develops a raised, red appearance. If this is over a joint, then it can cause flexion and ultimately the part will become contracted (Dealey, 2005). These patients should be referred to a burns unit for specialised care.

Non-healing acute wounds can become a chronic wound and be problematic to manage.

CHRONIC WOUNDS

Chronic wounds are a manifestation of various underlying problems and pathological conditions. The most frequently occurring chronic wounds are leg ulcers, pressure ulcers and diabetic foot ulcers. Other types of chronic wounds include non-healing surgical wounds, burns, malignant wounds and fistulae.

Holistic assessment of the patient is the keystone to management of chronic wounds. It is important to take concomitant medical conditions into consideration as they may cause delays in healing. Your practice should be supported by good evidence. It is therefore recommended that you follow evidence-based clinical guidelines, as discussed in the introductory chapter of this book. Their use has been demonstrated to be effective in improving patient outcomes (Bahtsevani *et al.*, 2004).

Pressure ulcers

Pressure ulcers are commonly found over bony prominences, especially the sacrum, buttocks and heels. Fig. 7.4 illustrates all the bony prominences on the body. Identification of early signs of pressure damage is essential to prevent extensive damage. It is generally considered that about 95% of pressure ulcers can be prevented (Hagisawa & Barbanel, 1999). The key to prevention is identification of those at risk of developing pressure ulcers and then developing an appropriate prevention strategy, such as given in the National Institute for Health and Clinical Excellence (NICE) guidelines on pressure ulcer risk assessment and prevention (NICE, 2001). An important aspect of prevention is to monitor the status of the skin in order to identify areas of persistent redness over a bony prominence, which is often the first indication of pressure damage. It may be possible to reverse the damage at this stage.

Further detail on the prevention of pressure ulcers is beyond the remit of this book; the rest of this section focuses on the management of existing pressure ulcers.

Assessment

When assessing a patient with a pressure ulcer the following factors should be considered:

• Why or how did the ulcer occur – what were the factors involved?

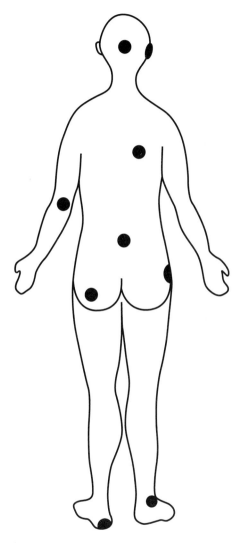

Fig. 7.4 The bony prominences.

- Factors relating to the development of the ulcer and their potential impact on healing.
- The extent of the damage.

Why or how did the ulcer occur – what were the factors involved?

When assessing a patient with a pressure ulcer it is essential to identify the specific cause of the ulcer and to remove that cause if possible. Pressure ulcers are generally caused by an episode of prolonged pressure over a bony prominence in a vulnerable person. Vulnerability to development of pressure ulcers is associated with immobility, loss of sensation, reduced tissue resilience, e.g. ageing skin, and incontinence. However, the precise circumstances will vary for each individual (see Box 7.1).

Assessing the extent of the damage

Pressure ulcers are generally described in terms relating to the depth of skin damage. This is known as pressure ulcer grading, and many different methods are in use. The commonest grading system in use in the UK is that developed by the European Pressure Ulcer Advisory Panel (EPUAP, 1999). This is described below and illustrated in Fig. 7.5.

- *Grade 1:* non-blanchable erythema of intact skin. Discoloration of the skin, warmth, oedema, induration or hardness may also be used as indicators, particularly on individuals with darker skin.
- *Grade 2:* partial thickness skin loss involving epidermis, dermis, or both. The ulcer is superficial and presents clinically as an abrasion or blister.

Box 7.1

Case history A

Mrs A is 83 years old and has become quite frail. When going to the toilet she tripped and fell, breaking her hip. She could not move and as a result became incontinent of urine. She was found by her daughter some hours later and taken to hospital. Following surgery to repair the hip fracture, Mrs A was found to have a pressure ulcer on her sacrum. The causes of this pressure ulcer were: pressure from lying on the hard floor; immobility; fragile skin because of her age and incontinence.

Case history B

Keith is a 23-year-old man with paraplegia who has a specially designed wheelchair and lives independently. He has a cushion in his wheelchair that provides pressure redistribution and assists in preventing pressure damage. The cushion had been provided by the wheelchair service 4 years ago and had not been assessed since that time as Keith had failed to attend his clinic appointments. He noticed some staining on his underwear and discovered that he had a pressure ulcer on his left buttock. The cause of the pressure ulcer was a result of prolonged pressure due to the worn out cushion, plus his immobility and loss of sensation due to paraplegia.

- *Grade 3:* full thickness skin loss involving damage to or necrosis of subcutaneous tissue that may extend down to, but not through, underlying fascia.
- *Grade 4:* extensive destruction, tissue necrosis, or damage to muscle, bone, or supporting structures with or without full thickness skin loss.

Grade 1   Grade 2

Grade 3   Grade 4

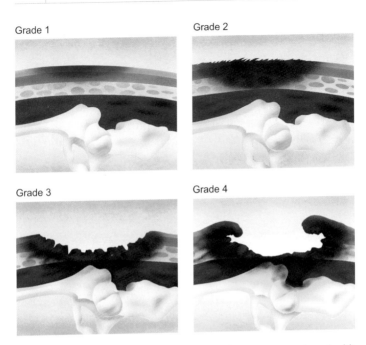

Fig. 7.5 EPUAP pressure ulcer grading. Images reproduced with kind permission from Huntleigh Healthcare Ltd.

In addition to determining the grade, an ulcer should also be assessed as any other wound as discussed in Chapter 5.

Management

A starting point for managing a pressure ulcer is to remove the cause wherever possible. For example, Mrs A in case history A in Box 7.1 would remain vulnerable to further pressure damage because of her frailty. However, the risk would reduce once she becomes mobile again. Keith's (case history B) pressure ulcer was directly caused by failure of his pressure redistributing cushion and it would need to be replaced. Keith will remain at long-term risk of developing pressure ulcers due to his immobility and loss of sensation caused by his paraplegia.

Relief of pressure

It is important to ensure that there is as little pressure as possible over the pressure ulcer to promote healing. Traditionally, this has been achieved by regular repositioning of the patient and is sometimes called '2 hourly turning'. The NICE guidelines for the prevention and treatment of pressure ulcers recommend that all patients with pressure ulcers should be encouraged to mobilise or change their position frequently and if they cannot do so themselves, they should be repositioned frequently (NICE, 2005). A repositioning schedule should be established, taking the patient's other activities into consideration (NICE, 2005). For example, bedfast patients should not be turned onto their sides during mealtimes, but sat up in order to be able to eat properly, even if for a very restricted time.

The other strategy for relief of pressure is to use pressure-redistributing devices.

Equipment

Many devices are available for pressure ulcer prevention including mattresses, overlays, specialised beds and cushions. They are made of a variety of materials and work by either reducing pressure or relieving pressure. Pressure reduction occurs when the patient 'sinks' into a device, thus spreading the weight load and reducing the pressure over the bony prominences. Pressure relief is achieved by removal of pressure over a bony prominence in a cyclical manner. Table 7.2 provides details of the common types of mattresses and overlays. The NICE guidelines recommend that patients with grade 1 or 2 pressure ulcers should, as a minimum, be placed on a high-specification foam mattress or cushion (NICE, 2005). Patients with grade 3 or 4 pressure ulcers are likely to need a more sophisticated device such as alternating air mattresses or overlays. Selection of an appropriate device will depend on a range of factors such as overall health status, level of mobility, patient acceptability and lifestyle. The tissue viability nurse may be involved in selecting suitable devices for patients with complex problems. Some trusts may have an equipment store to provide, monitor and maintain equipment and to

Table 7.2 Types of pressure redistributing equipment.

Category	Type of equipment	Bed	Mattress	Overlay
'Low tech' devices	High-specification foam		✓	✓
	Cut foam		✓	✓
	Gel-filled		✓	✓
	Fluid-filled		✓	✓
	Air-filled		✓	✓
'High tech' devices	Alternating pressure		✓	✓
	Low air loss	✓	✓	✓
	Air fluidised	✓		
	Turning beds	✓		

ensure that there is 24-hour access to pressure redistributing devices.

Nutrition

The importance of nutrition in wound healing has already been discussed in Chapter 3. All patients with pressure ulcers should have their nutritional status assessed which should include regular weighing of patients, skin assessment, documentation of food and fluid intake (EPUAP, 2003). If it is not possible to improve the patient's intake of food and fluids, nutritional supplementation may be considered (EPUAP, 2003).

Local wound care

As with any other wound, pressure ulcers need to be assessed and appropriate treatment goals set (see Chapter 5). However, deep pressure ulcers are often associated with necrotic tissue which must be debrided before the wound can heal. As the necrotic tissue liquefies, the wound may produce a foul-smelling heavy exudate. This should not be mistaken for infection, although obviously if there are clinical signs of infection they should not be ignored. Patients need to understand what is happening as they may find this phase distressing. NICE recommends that progress towards healing should be reviewed weekly and that the pressure ulcer grade, size and appearance should be recorded (NICE, 2005). It should always be remembered that however appropriate the dressing selection for a pressure ulcer may be, it will not be effective if there is inadequate pressure relief.

Leg ulcers

Assessment

Leg ulcers occur most commonly in association with venous and/or arterial disease. The holistic management of a patient with a leg ulcer is determined by the outcome of the assessment. Therefore only a competent practitioner should undertake the assessment, which should include an assessment of the health of the patient, the underlying aetiology of the ulcer and local wound and skin conditions. Many patients are elderly and have co-existing medical conditions such as diabetes, rheumatoid arthritis, cardiac problems, poor mobility and other factors that can influence treatment and affect healing. The impact of the ulcer on the patient's quality of life should be considered (see Chapter 9 for further details).

Patients have found pain to be an overwhelming feature of both venous and arterial ulceration and this should be documented and a pain management plan instigated (discussed in Chapter 8). Hand-held Doppler ultrasound is used to establish whether there is an adequate blood supply to the limb. This is a non-invasive screening test that determines the degree of arterial insufficiency in an ulcerated limb. The technique consists of measuring the systolic blood pressure in the arm and the ankle, with the patient lying down on a bed or couch, then dividing the ankle pressure by the arm pressure (Table 7.3). The result is termed as the ankle/brachial pressure index (ABPI). Only a person who has been suitably trained in this procedure should undertake the ABPI measurement and interpret the results.

Table 7.3 Ankle brachial pressure index (ABPI).

$ABPI = \dfrac{\text{ankle systolic pressure}}{\text{brachial systolic pressure}}$	With patient lying on bed or couch
ABPI > 1.0	Indicates normal arterial blood supply
ABPI 0.8–0.95	Indicates some arterial impairment
ABPI < 0.8	Indicates significant arterial impairment

VENOUS LEG ULCERATION

A venous leg ulcer is a wound on the lower leg that has occurred or failed to heal due to incompetent valves in the veins. The venous system of the leg consists of the deep veins, superficial veins, perforator veins and one-way valves. These components work together with the calf muscles to pump blood back to the heart against the force of gravity (Burnand & Browse, 1982). Veins have one-way valves that allow blood to flow in one direction, i.e. towards the heart. Failure of these 'one-way' valves in the deep and perforating veins allows backflow of blood from the deep veins to the superficial veins which become stretched and dilated, leading to damage to other valves that were previously competent. This causes abnormally high pressure in the superficial veins, known as venous hypertension, and leads to a rise in pressure in the capillaries and subsequent leakage of red blood cells into the tissue spaces. However, the precise mechanism by which venous hypertension results in leg ulceration remains unclear. Research suggests that many pathological processes may be involved (Burnand *et al.*, 1982; Coleridge-Smith *et al.*, 1988; Thomas *et al.*, 1988; Falanga & Eaglstein, 1993).

Clinical signs

- *Brown staining* is seen in the skin above the medial malleolus, caused by breakdown of red blood cells and deposition of haemosiderin.
- *Oedema* is often a feature of venous disease, where high pressure in the capillaries causes leakage of fluid into the tissues.
- *Varicose eczema* is often present on the lower leg of a patient with a venous leg ulcer.

Management

Following the assessment each patient should have an individualised plan of care, based on a clear rational for the desired outcome as explained here. If the ulcer is deemed to be venous in aetiology then conservative treatment will be with compression therapy, elevation and exercise. It is now widely accepted that compression is the most important factor in the treatment of venous leg ulcers (Effective Health Care Bulletin, 1997; Fletcher *et al.*, 1997), and many compression bandaging systems are available. It is essential that a compression bandage is applied only by a practitioner who has been trained to do. Failure to apply the bandage correctly could lead to serious tissue damage.

Local wound care

The wound and surrounding skin should be assessed to determine the most suitable appropriate primary dressing as discussed in Chapters 4 and 5. The peri-wound skin should be protected from wound exudate as discussed in Chapter 6. Skin can be kept moisturised with a simple emollient such as 50% white soft paraffin in 50% liquid paraffin (50/50). If a patient has cellulitis (see Chapter 5), then the compression bandage should be discontinued and only used once the infection has settled.

ARTERIAL ULCERS

Arterial ulcers occur because of reduced arterial blood supply, resulting in tissue ischaemia and necrosis. They are more common in people who smoke, have diabetes and in older people (Holloway, 2001). Patients may complain of pain in their leg when walking (intermittent claudication), indicating an inadequate blood supply to the painful area during exercise, or they may have pain even when the limb is at rest (Holloway, 2001). Measurement of the ABPI, as described above, will determine the degree of arterial insufficiency in the limb (see Table 7.3).

Management

Smoking exacerbates the condition and patients should be strongly advised to stop. Patients with arterial disease will require specialist interventions such as surgery or angioplasty to improve the blood supply. Patients with an impaired arterial blood supply should not have compression applied to the limb or high elevation. A light retention bandage, such as a cotton non-elastic tubular bandage, is all that is required to hold dressings or padding in place.

Local wound care

The wound should be kept moist and any necrotic tissue and slough removed. This may be achieved by autolytic debridement facilitated by dressings that rehydrate the wound, such as hydrogels and hydrocolloids, or by bio-surgery (larvae therapy) (see Chapter 4 for more information on dressing selection). Dressings applied to an arterial ulcer will not improve healing until an adequate blood supply has been achieved following surgical intervention (Holloway, 2001).

DIABETIC FOOT ULCERS

The most commonly occurring diabetic foot ulcers are those associated with peripheral neuropathy (nerve damage), peripheral vascular disease (poor blood supply) and deformity (Jude *et al.*, 2001; Steed, 2001). Deformity may lead to increased foot pressures and ulceration.

Management

The main goal is to prevent the occurrence of a diabetic foot ulcer. Patients with diabetes should be encouraged to inspect their feet daily for any changes to their normal skin tissue such as reddening, blisters and areas of dry hardened skin. If the patient is ill in hospital then the nurse responsible for their holistic care should undertake this.

Local wound care

If foot ulceration or new areas of inflammation should occur, the patient should be referred for urgent expert assessment. Management of a diabetic foot ulcer requires a team approach to care. The hospital or community podiatrist, the diabetic nurse specialist or the diabetic foot clinic team are valuable resources who can provide expert advice on the management of a patient with a diabetic foot ulcer. A podiatrist can provide devices such as felt inserts, orthopaedic shoes or diabetic walkers to relieve any pressure and improve healing prospects (King, 2002). Appropriate referral and treatment is essential as failure to manage a diabetic ulcer appropriately can lead to gangrene and amputation (Steed, 2001).

Key points

- Healing with the skin edges closed is called healing by primary intention.
- Healing by secondary intention is when there is tissue loss and the skin edges are far apart and the wound heals from the base upwards.
- The commonest complications of surgical wounds are haemorrhage, infection and dehiscence (breakdown of the suture line).
- Patients should be given clear information prior to surgery, so that they know what to expect.
- Simple lacerations can be managed conservatively whereas severe lacerations may require surgery.
- Traumatic wounds are likely to be heavily contaminated with bacteria and so are at great risk of infection.
- The spread of a burn injury is measured in terms of the percentage of the body surface area that is affected.
- Medical assistance is required immediately for anyone with a major burn.
- However appropriate the dressing selection for any of the wounds described in this chapter may be, it will not

Continued

be effective if the underlying cause has not been addressed.

- The key to pressure ulcer prevention is identifying at-risk patients and implementing an appropriate prevention strategy.
- Pressure ulcers are commonly found over bony prominences *and* are generally described in terms relating to the depth of skin damage.
- An important part of pressure ulcer management is to remove the cause wherever possible.
- A venous leg ulcer is a wound on the lower leg that has occurred or failed to heal due to incompetent valves in the veins.
- Compression is the most important factor in the treatment of venous leg ulcers and should only be applied by a practitioner who has been trained to do so.
- Patients with arterial disease will require specialist interventions such as surgery or angioplasty to improve their blood supply.
- Patients with diabetes should be encouraged to inspect their feet daily as part of a prevention strategy in the occurrence of a diabetic foot ulcer.
- Failure to manage a diabetic ulcer can lead to gangrene and amputation.
- All patients with a wound should have an assessment of the level of any pain they may be experiencing to ensure appropriate analgesia is given.

SUMMARY

This chapter has discussed the assessment and management of some of the most frequently occurring acute and chronic wounds. It should be read in conjunction with Chapters 4–6, which cover general assessment and

Continued

management of wounds and the peri-ulcer skin and developing a plan of care. You should now use the knowledge you have gained from reading these chapters to undertake the following exercise.

Exercise 7.1

Case scenario

Mrs Rosalind Barrett is a 78-year-old woman who has an ulcer on her left heel (see Fig. 7.6). The ulcer has been present for several weeks. Mrs Barrett has mild diabetes managed by diet alone. She is married and lives with her husband, who is the same age as her. They have a daughter, Elaine, who lives near by and helps them with their shopping and washing. Mr Barrett looks after their

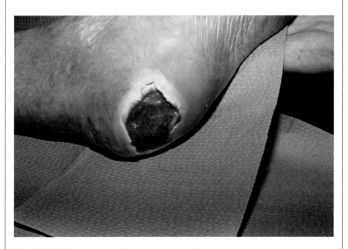

Fig. 7.6 Case scenario: pressure ulcer.

Continued

small garden and Mrs Barrett still does most of the cooking. They do not go out much as they both have failing eyesight. Mrs Barrett likes to spend time sitting and listening to music. She often goes barefoot in the house. Their kitchen has a tiled floor and the lounge has wood flooring with a rug in the centre. Mrs Barrett has always sat in an upright chair but is tending to spend a lot longer in the chair than she used to and this makes her back ache. To alleviate this she puts a cushion in her back, but now finds she constantly slips down and pushes herself up again by pressing down on her left heel. When collecting the washing Elaine noticed that there was staining on the lower part of the bed sheets and on the heel of her mother's stockings. Her mother insisted there was nothing wrong with her feet and that she must have got her foot wet while walking around in just her stockings. Elaine did not pursue it further. However, the staining was there again the next week. Elaine persuaded her mother to let her look at her feet and was surprised to see the skin on her left heel was broken and discharging. She dressed the wound herself with an Elastoplast dressing and suggested to her mother that if it did not improve she should see the practice nurse. Elaine was due to go on holiday the next day and a neighbour offered to do the washing. When Elaine returned after 2 weeks she had forgotten about her mother's heel and it was another week before she remembered and asked to see her heel again. Elaine was very alarmed by the appearance of the wound and made an immediate appointment for her mother to see the practice nurse at their local GP surgery.

Use a systematic approach to help you to determine what has caused Mrs Barrett's ulcer, what treatment to instigate and who will be involved in her care.

Continued

Step 1: assess the patient, wound and circumstances

Your assessment of Mrs Barrett should include her general health and any concomitant medical conditions, as these may increase risk factors and influence treatment decisions. You should look at her lifestyle as this may give you clues as to the development of the ulcer. When assessing the wound you should consider its position, appearance of the wound bed and what the surrounding skin looks like. You should establish Mrs Barrett's own perceptions of her wound. Your assessment may identify potential risk factors that need to be addressed.

Step 2: utilise existing information about the patient

You already know that Mrs Barrett has diabetes and has failing eyesight. She also likes to go barefoot in her house and will therefore have spent time standing on her kitchen floor doing the cooking as well as putting pressure on her heel when she slips in her chair. Think how these factors may have affected the development of this ulcer. You should establish who is monitoring her diabetes and when was the last time Mrs Barrett had an assessment. Who else is involved in her care?

Step 3: explore relevant current best practice

Consider who will be the most appropriate person to give good advice on best practice in the management of Mrs Barrett's heel ulcer.

Step 4: make a clinical decision

Following the assessment you should have enough information to enable you to determine what has caused this ulcer and the appropriate management of the patient, the

Continued

wound and peri-ulcer skin. Remember that however appropriate your dressing selection is for the wound state, it will not be effective if the underlying cause is not addressed.

Step 5: evaluate progress
Think about how you will re-assess the ulcer and what you will be looking for to evaluate whether the dressing regimen is effective.

Suggested management

Mrs Barrett has a pressure ulcer on her heel caused by her constantly pushing her bare heel on a hard surface. Mrs Barrett cannot feel pain in her heel and is therefore unaware that she has an ulcer on her heel. She also has diabetes and diabetic foot ulcers are commonly associated with peripheral neuropathy (nerve damage). Mrs Barrett should be referred for an urgent medical assessment of her diabetic status.

A starting point for managing Mrs Barrett's pressure ulcer is to remove the cause, which involves finding her suitable seating and appropriate foot wear. Management of a diabetic foot ulcer requires a team approach to care. The community podiatrist would be able to give advice on management and provide devices to relieve pressure over Mrs Barrett's ulcer, to improve her healing prospects. The wound is healthy and granulating but the surrounding skin is macerated (white maceration) where wound fluid has stayed in contact on the skin within her stocking. A suitable dressing regimen for the wound would be to apply an alginate dressing to the wound and a skin protectant such as zinc paste to the surrounding skin, a light pad and secure with tubular stockinette. The wound should be photographed and measured as a baseline to monitor progress. Once the pressure has been removed the wound should start to heal.

CONCLUSION

This exercise has shown you how to use a systematic approach to assessing and developing a plan of care for a patient with a diabetic foot ulcer.

REFERENCES

Alsbjörn, B., Gilbert, P., Hartmann, B., Kaźmierski, M., Monstrey, S., Palao, R., Roberto, M.A., van Trier, A. & Voinchey, V. (2007) Guidelines for the management of partial-thickness burns in a general hospital or community setting – recommendations of a European working party. *Burns* **33**: 155–160.

Bahtsevani, C., Uden, G. & Willman, A. (2004) Outcomes of evidence-based clinical practice guidelines: a systematic review. *International Journal of Technology Assessment in Health Care* **20**(4): 427–433.

Birchall, L. & Taylor, S. (2003) Surgical wound benchmark tool and best practice guidelines. *British Journal of Nursing* **12**(17): 1013–1023.

Briggs, M. (1996) Surgical wound pain: a trial of two treatments. *Journal of Wound Care* **5**(10): 456–460.

Burnand, K. & Browse, N.L. (1982) The post phlebitic leg and venous ulceration. In: Russell, R.C.G. (ed) *Recent Advances in Surgery* **11**. Edinburgh, Churchill Livingstone.

Burnand, K., Whimster, I. & Naidoo, A. (1982) Pericapillary fibrin in the ulcer bearing skin of the leg: the cause of lipodermatosclerosis and venous ulceration. *British Medical Journal* **285**: 1920–1922.

Coleridge-Smith, P., Thomas, P., Scurr, J.H. & Dormandy, J.A. (1988) Causes of venous ulceration: a new hypothesis. *British Medical Journal* **296**: 1726–1727.

Dealey, C. (2005) *The Care of Wounds, Third Edition*. Oxford, Blackwell Science.

Dunkin, C.S.J., Elfleet, D., Ling, C. & Brown, T.P.L.H. (2003) A step-by-step guide to classifying and managing pretibial lacerations. *Journal of Wound Care* **12**(3): 109–112.

Effective Health Care Bulletin (1997) Compression therapy for venous leg ulcers. University of York, NHS Centre for Reviews and Dissemination.

Emmerson, A.M., Enstone, J.E., Griffin, M., Kelsey, M.C. & Smyth, E.T. (1996) The second national prevalence survey of infection in hospitals – overview of the results. *Journal of Hospital Infection* **32:** 175–190.

European Pressure Ulcer Advisory Panel (1999) Pressure ulcer treatment guidelines. *EPUAP Review* **1**(2): 31–33.

European Pressure Ulcer Advisory Panel (2003) *Nutritional Guidelines for Pressure Ulcer Prevention and Treatment*. Oxford, EPUAP.

Falanga, V. & Eaglstein, W.H. (1993) The trap hypothesis of venous ulceration. *Lancet* **341**: 1006–1008.

Farion, K., Osmond, M.H., Hartling, L. *et al.* (2004) Tissue adhesives for trauma lacerations in children and adults (Cochrane review). *Cochrane Library*, Issue 4. Chichester, John Wiley & Sons Ltd.

Fletcher, A., Cullum, N. & Sheldon, T.A. (1997) A systematic review of compression treatment for venous leg ulcers. *British Medical Journal* **315**: 576–580.

Hagisawa, S. & Barbanel, J. (1999) The limits of pressure sore prevention. *Journal of the Royal Society of Medicine* **92**(11): 576–578.

Holloway, G.A. Jr. (2001) Arterial ulcers: assessment, classification and management. In: Krasner, D.L., Rodeheaver, G.T. & Sibbald, R.G. (eds) *Chronic Wound*

Care: A Clinical Source Book for Healthcare Professionals, Third Edition. Wayne, PA, HMP Communications.

Jude, E., Armstrong, D.G. & Boulton, A.J.M. (2001) Assessment of the diabetic foot. In: Krasner, D.L., Rodeheaver, G.T. & Sibbald, R.G. (eds) Chronic Wound Care: A Clinical Source Book for Healthcare Professionals, Third Edition. Wayne, PA, HMP Communications, pp. 589–597.

King, L. (2002) Assessment and management of the diabetic foot. In: Cherry, G. (ed) The Oxford European Wound Healing Course Handbook. Oxford, Positif Press, pp. 62–68.

Mangram, A.J., Horan, T.C., Pearson, M.L., Silver, L.C. & Jarvis, W.R. (1999) Guideline for the prevention of SSI. Infection Control and Epidemiology 20(4): 267–278.

National Institute for Clinical Excellence (2001) Pressure Ulcer Risk Assessment and Prevention. London, NICE.

National Institute for Health and Clinical Excellence and the Royal College of Nursing (2005). The Management of Pressure Ulcers in Primary and Secondary Care. London, NICE.

Prodigy Guidance (2004) Burns and scalds. CKS Library. Available at: http://cks.library.nhs.uk/burns_and_scalds/print (accessed 12 Aug 2007).

Ratcliffe, C.R. & Fletcher, K.R. (2007) Skin tear: a review of the evidence to support prevention and treatment. Ostomy and Wound Management 53(3): 32–42.

Reg, R. & Johnson, R.M. (2002) Managing superficial burn wounds. Advances in Skin and Wound Care 15(5): 246–247.

Sargent, R.L. (2006) Management of blisters in the partial-thickness burn: an integrative research review. Journal of Burn Care and Research 27(1): 66–81.

Small, V. (2000) Management of cuts, abrasions and lacerations. Nursing Standard 15(5): 41–44.

St John's Ambulance (2007) Burns and scalds. Available at: http://www.sja.org.uk/first-aid-advice/effects-of-heat-and-cold/burns-and-scalds.aspx (accessed 29 July 2007).

Steed, D.L. (2001) Diabetic wounds: assessment, classification and management. In: Krasner, D.L., Rodeheaver, G.T. & Sibbald, R.G. (eds) *Chronic Wound Care: A Clinical Source Book for Healthcare Professionals, Third Edition*. Wayne, PA, HMP Communications, pp. 575–581.

Thomas, P.R., Nash, G.B. & Dormandy, J.A. (1988) White cell accumulation in dependent legs of patients with venous hypertension: a possible mechanism for trophic changes in the skin. *British Medical Journal* **296**: 507–509.

Wallace, A.B. (1951) The exposure treatment of burns. *Lancet* **1**: 501–504.

Watret, L. & White, R. (2001) Surgical wound management: the role of dressings. *Nursing Standard* **15**(44): 59–69.

Pain

8

Deborah Hofman

INTRODUCTION

Pain is a major concern for most patients with wounds and is often poorly and inadequately managed. However, in recent years there has been an increasing interest and awareness of the problem. Wound pain may be caused by the initial trauma that resulted in the wound or persistent trauma to the wound bed, or it may be due to the underlying disease process that caused the wound. It may be also associated with interventions such as debridement (removal of dead tissue from the wound bed) or dressing changes.

This chapter will consider reasons why pain is an important aspect of wound management and why it is often mismanaged by practitioners, and provide an overview of the physiology of pain, describe how to assess a patient suffering from wound-related pain, and discuss ways in which wound-related pain can be most effectively managed.

WHY IS THE EFFECTIVE MANAGEMENT OF WOUND-RELATED PAIN IMPORTANT?

Pain associated with wounds should be as important to the practitioner as it is to the patient. Not only does continuous pain have an obvious negative impact on quality of life but it can also affect clinical outcomes and impair wound healing. Patients in pain experience a variety of physiological changes that can be detrimental to their health such as increased blood pressure, altered blood gases, delayed gastric emptying or urinary retention (Johnson, 2006). High levels of pain cause psychological stress, which in turn has been shown to be detrimental to wound healing (Kiecolt–Glaser *et al.*, 1995; McGuire *et al.*, 2006). Emotions such as fear, anger, depression, can influence pain perception. In addition, healing may be impaired by sleep

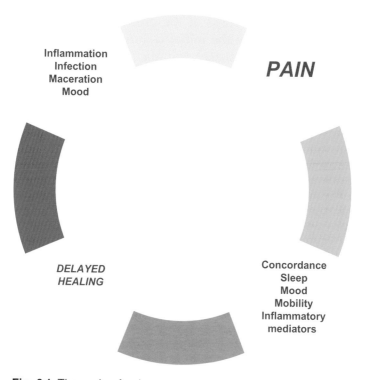

Inflammation
Infection
Maceration
Mood

PAIN

*DELAYED
HEALING*

Concordance
Sleep
Mood
Mobility
Inflammatory
mediators

Fig. 8.1 The cycle of pain.

deprivation, heightened stress levels, immobility and increased inflammation caused by pain. Patients may be unable to comply with treatment such as compression bandaging, due to pain. Moreover, a wound that fails to heal is at risk of becoming infected, leading to further delayed healing and further associated depression so that a vicious circle of pain and non-healing can occur (Fig. 8.1). Successful interventions to lessen pain will not only improve quality of life but also improve the overall health of the patient and in many cases expedite wound healing.

WHY IS WOUND PAIN OFTEN POORLY MANAGED?

There is often an inadequate understanding about the importance of pain on the part of practitioners. This may be due to several reasons.

- Practitioners are often so focused on treating the wound that they forget that the patient is in pain.
- Pain is seen to be a normal part of having a wound and therefore not addressed (Ready & Edwards, 1992).
- There may be reluctance to give analgesia due to concern about side effects and misplaced fear of addiction.
- Patients tend not to report pain unless asked and many practitioners do not ask.

WHAT IS PAIN?

The International Association for the Study of Pain (ISAP) defines pain as: 'an unpleasant sensory and emotional experience associated with actual or potential tissue damage, or described in terms of such damage' (Merskey & Bogduk, 1994). This definition indicates that pain is not only a sensory phenomenon but that also a patient's emotions have a large impact on pain perception. The reverse is also true, insofar as a patient who is in pain may also become affected emotionally and become depressed, angry or fearful. This definition also implies that though chronic pain is usually associated with tissue damage this is not always the case (for example phantom limb pain). The definition describes how patients often use terms associated with tissue damage to describe their pain, for example 'stabbing', 'burning' 'cutting'.

Another description of pain is that proposed by McCaffery (1983): 'Pain is whatever the patient says it is and occurs whenever the patient says it does'. This statement emphasises that pain is subjective and that only patients can describe their pain and its impact on their life. However, sometimes patients are reluctant or unable to discuss their pain. It may be true that patients sometimes have need to exaggerate their pain but it is very difficult for practitioners to assess this accurately or to understand the underlying motives and it is a dangerous conclusion to make. It is extremely demoralising and distressing for a patient not to have their pain believed and this can erode the trust between practitioner and patient.

PHYSIOLOGY OF NORMAL PAIN

The body's nervous system specifically dedicated to detecting pain is known as the nociceptive system. It consists of:

- *Nociceptors (sensation)*: these are sensory receptors in the skin that are sensitive to noxious or painful stimuli or to stimuli which would become painful if prolonged.
- *Neural pathways (transmission)*: these consist of A and C fibres that send nerve impulses to the central nervous system (spinal cord and brain).
- *Processing areas (perception)*: these are neural areas in the brain that process incoming impulses to generate an awareness of the painful stimuli via the sensation of pain and interpret pain, identifying its cause and effect on the body. Emotional response to pain is generated in the brain.

GATE THEORY AND DIMENSIONS OF PAIN

As previously stated in this chapter, pain is not only a physiological response to tissue damage but its perception can be altered by emotion and experience. In 1965 Ronald Melzack (a psychologist) and Patrick Wall (an anatomist) worked together and presented the 'gate control theory' of pain (Melzack & Wall, 1965). This theory postulates that a metaphorical gate in the spinal cord regulates the flow of noxious information on its way to the brain. If the gate is open, noxious information can reach the brain to generate the sensation of pain. If the gate is closed noxious information cannot reach the brain and the sensation of pain does not result. Transmission through the gate depends not only on the intensity of the peripheral stimulus but also on other competing stimuli and descending impulses higher up in the nervous system. This explains why distraction techniques can help reduce pain perception. Further work in this area suggested there are distinct dimensions of pain perception (Melzack & Wall, 1988).

- *Sensory dimension*: relates to the intensity, location and quality of pain. Information is provided by the nociceptive system and is then relayed to and from the cortex of the brain.
- *Affective dimension*: relates to the emotional aspects of pain. Information is provided by the nociceptive system and is modified in the brain. For example, a patient who is very frightened may experience higher levels of pain.

These models of pain perception illustrate that pain is not exclusively sensory and that simple measures of pain intensity are inadequate to understand it.

DURATION OF PAIN
Acute pain
Acute pain can be defined as pain of limited duration and usually has causal relationship to injury and disease. It may be of 'brief duration and of little consequence' (Melzack & Wall, 1988) apart from being a learning experience in avoiding such injury in the future and aiding tissue repair by making the injured area more sensitive and thus preventing further injury. The consequence of absence of this response can be seen in patients with absence of sensation in their feet associated with diabetes, which can lead to catastrophic injuries. Acute pain may also signify that there is a deterioration in the wound, due to infection, ischaemia, injury (this may be iatrogenic, i.e. caused by the practitioner) or inflammation, which may need

Table 8.1 Useful pain (the 4 Is).

Infection	Check for other signs of infection
Inflammation	May be associated with infection
Ischaemia	Leg ulcer: check foot pulses and Doppler (as described in Chapter 7)
	Check wound margins for signs of bluish discoloration
	Ensure there is no pressure on the wound
Iatrogenic (injury caused by practitioner)	Reassess appropriateness of dressing and that bandages are correctly applied

Adapted with permission from Hofman (2006b).

prompt intervention. Pain should be regarded as the fifth vital sign (Turk & Melzack, 2001) (along with temperature, pulse, blood pressure, and respiration rate), and its presence should never be ignored either in an acute surgical wound or in a chronic wound (see Table 8.1).

Chronic pain (persistent pain)

Chronic pain is pain associated with an injury which is not resolved within an expected period of time, for example pain associated with a chronic wound or an ongoing disease process such as cancer or an ischaemic limb. It may manifest itself as recurrent episodes of acute pain. Persistent pain may be associated with ongoing tissue damage as in chronic wounds and can be divided into two categories:

- *Useful pain*: this acts as a warning signal that something is going wrong in the wound, i.e. infection, ischaemia, injury or inflammation. Increased pain levels post surgery may also be a symptom of bleeding into the tissues.
- *Useless pain*: this is where the nociceptive system has become sensitised, damaged and dysfunctional (neuropathic pain). Neuropathic pain can be characterised by unusual symptoms such as numbness, shooting pains, electrical sensations and deep aching. In addition the signs *hyperalgesia* or *allodynia* as described below may be present. An understanding of these types of abnormal pain sensations will have an impact on a nurse's appreciation of a patient's pain during dressing change.

Hyperalgesia
In hyperalgesia pain sensation is exaggerated either within the wound or in the healthy tissue surrounding the wound. This type of pain may cause a patient to cry out in pain when lightly touched during dressing change.

Allodynia
Allodynia means that non-noxious stimuli, for example light touch, are perceived as painful either in or around the wound. Neuropathic pain has no benefit in terms of protecting the wound from further damage in contrast with nociceptive pain.

ASSESSMENT

'Just as my pain belongs in a unique way only to me, so I am utterly alone with it. I cannot share it' (Illich, 1976).

'To understand and adequately treat pain we have to be able to measure it' (Turk & Melzack, 2001).

Pain assessment in patients with wounds is a complex procedure and requires time and thought. Establishing the cause of the pain is of vital importance in order to identify the cause of the symptoms and suggest a course of management. The nurse must be clear as to what is causing the wound as well as what may be causing the pain within the wound. In the case of a surgical wound increase in pain in conjunction with raised temperature and pulse rate may suggest infection. In a chronic wound that becomes infected there may be little in the way of clinical signs and the only clue may be pain or increased pain.

Leg ulcer pain is particularly complex (Hofman, 2006a) and the pain is often related to the aetiology of the wound. Pain assessment should be incorporated into every leg ulcer assessment and should be carried out by a suitably trained nurse. It may be that interventions such as dressing change or debridement are either exacerbating or causing the pain. If this is the case then pain prevention strategies should be clearly identified while planning care.

Key factors in assessment

Six key factors are commonly identified as the basic essentials of all pain assessment (McCaffery & Pasero, 1999; Dunn, 2000).

- *Location*: in the wound, around the wound, referred elsewhere.
- *Description*: ask patient to describe pain in their own words.

- *Duration*: how long has the pain been present?
- *Intensity*: how bad is the pain? A formal assessment tool (see below) may be used.
- *Influencing factors*: factors that either help relieve pain, for example position, movement, or aggravate the pain, for example dressing change.
- *Previous treatment*: what has or has not worked. What analgesia is the patient taking and has it made any difference? Have any dressings made the pain better/worse?

PAIN SCALES

There is no consensus on a single method of assessing a patient in pain and many competing instruments, procedures and methods are available. The most important question to be asked is, 'Are you in pain and if so tell me where it hurts?'. Having established that the patient is in pain, a suitable pain scale can be selected to assess severity.

Commonly used pain scales are:

- Verbal Rating Scale (VRS): this scale consists of a range of words from no pain to unbearable pain. The words to describe the pain may be predetermined or the patient's own words may be used.
- Numerical Scale: patients are asked to describe their pain in numbers rather words. For example from 0 = no pain to 10 = the worst possible pain.
- Visual Analogue Scale (VAS): patients are asked to indicate the intensity of their pain by placing a mark on a line with no pain at one end and unbearable pain at the other. Figure 8.2 is an example of a combination of a VRS and VAS scale.

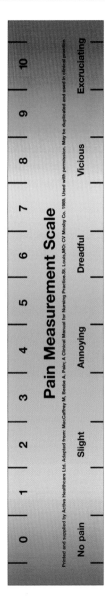

Fig. 8.2 Example of a combination of a VRS and VAS scale. Reproduced with kind permission from Activa Healthcare Ltd.

- Faces Rating Scale: This scale represents the intensity of pain using faces from a continuum from smiling to crying. These can be useful for children or in adults who have difficulty in conceptualising pain as a number or a word.

These pain scales can be used to assess a patient's overall pain or to assess pain at an intervention, for example dressing change and also ongoing assessment. Unfortunately research shows that few nurses use scales in assessing pain, preferring to use subjective judgements (McCaffery *et al.*, 2000; Briggs, 2006). The problem with the latter approach is that research has shown that nurses tend to underestimate patients' pain (Moffatt *et al.*, 2002; Briggs, 2006) and patients will suffer as a result.

MANAGING WOUND-RELATED PAIN
Pain at dressing changes

Pain at dressing changes can be difficult to avoid and the topic has been covered in two consensus documents (European Wound Management Association (EWMA), 2002; World Union of Wound Healing Societies (WUWHS) 2004). A previous negative experience will have an impact on the patient's pain perception so it is essential to build a good rapport with patients. Reassurance and creating a relaxed atmosphere is also important. The patient may prefer to remove their own dressing. Distraction techniques such as having someone else there to talk to the patient may be helpful. In severe cases systemic analgesia may be administered prior to the procedure or gas and oxygen may be given. Analgesic lozenges, although expensive, are very effective and user friendly. However, in most cases selection of a non-adherent dressing is sufficient to allow for pain-free dressing changes. Traditional dressings such as gauze and paraffin gauze often cause pain and trauma on dressing removal and should be avoided (WUWHS, 2004). Some modern adhesive backed dressings may cause trauma to fragile skin and sometimes to the wound bed (Hollinworth, 2005). However, soft silicone dressings do not adhere either to the wound bed or to the surrounding skin and may be safely left in place for up to 7 days.

Tissue injury
Tissue injury may occur if the dressing has been badly positioned or a bandage has not been applied correctly and consequently is cutting into the skin and cause unnecessary pain and distress to the patient.

Impact of exudate
If a moist dressing is applied to a heavily exuding wound, maceration and wound extension is likely to occur causing pain. Conversely a dry dressing on a dry wound will cause tissue adherence and pain. Maintaining optimal moisture balance at the wound interface by judicious choice of dressings is crucial for patient comfort as well as enhancing wound healing. See Chapter 4 for further information on the use of dressings.

Infection
The signs of infection (heat, redness, pain and swelling) have previously been discussed in Chapter 5.

However the first sign of high bacterial loads in a wound bed is often increased pain, with odour and increased exudate. There are at present different categories of dressings available for treating wounds that are heavily colonised with bacteria. Cadexomer iodine dressings have been available for many years, and more recently honey and silver dressings have become popular. They all have a role, but unfortunately many patients find the honey and iodine dressings very painful after application. See Chapter 4 for further information on the use of dressings.

Pain at debridement
Sharp debridement should only be undertaken by a suitably qualified practitioner. The nurse looking after the patient should ensure that the procedure is not painful for the patient. Application of topical local anaesthetic can be effective. Patients must be reassured that the procedure will stop if they so request.

Persistent pain
Persistent pain is continual ongoing pain. There are dressings now available that have been shown to relieve pain in many patients. These are recent innovations in the realms of wound care enabling nurses to make a substantial difference to their patients' well-being. Specialist nurses may be available to advise you on their use. However, in many cases pain is not controllable by dressings alone and appropriate analgesia should be prescribed. It should be remembered that any drug can give a patient unpleasant side effects and if this occurs another drug should be considered.

Key points

- Understanding the basics of the physiology of pain enables the practitioner to assess pain.
- Assessment of pain is necessary in order to treat pain.
- Wound pain should never be ignored because of the distress/discomfort caused to patients and because pain may be symptomatic of wound deterioration.
- In many cases wound pain may be managed by use of appropriate dressings.
- Sufficient, appropriate and timely analgesia should be given.

SUMMARY

This chapter has focused on giving you a basic understanding of the pathophysiology of pain, an understanding of the importance of pain assessment, the tools which are available to help you assess pain and some guidance on the management of wound-related pain. You should be aware that you may not always succeed in alleviating pain associated with wounds but it is important to make the patient aware that you consider their pain a problem and that you will continue trying to find measures to treat the pain. Seek help from specialists in the field (pain clinics, clinical nurse specialists) if you need further assistance.

You should now use the knowledge you have gained from reading this chapter to undertake the following exercise.

Exercise 8.1

Case scenario

Ken Ridgmore is a 68-year-old man who has a painful, dehisced surgical wound in his left groin. He has recently had vascular surgery, and 1 week post surgery the wound in his groin dehisced. Ken is a slightly built man who has dry, fragile, 'papery' skin and a decision has been made to allow his wound to heal by secondary intention. Ken is having difficulty walking, as his wound is painful and his dressing adheres to the wound and the securing tape pulls. Ken has been prescribed regular analgesia that is managing to keep his pain under control, but he still finds having his dressing changed very painful. Ken is due to have his dressing changed today and is very anxious.

Using a systematic approach, consider how you will reassure Ken and endeavour to make his dressing change as pain free as possible.

Step 1: assess the patient, wound and circumstances
You should consider how you will assess Ken's pain, the position of his wound, why his dressing is adhering to the wound, what may be contributing or causing his pain at dressing changes and what his main concerns are.

Step 2: utilise existing information about the patient
You should take into consideration that: Ken has very fragile skin; this wound has affected his mobility; he is taking regular analgesia; he finds dressing changes painful; and he is very anxious.

Continued

Step 3: explore relevant current best practice
You should consider what types of dressings are recommended to avoid adherence and when would be the most appropriate time to undertake the dressing.

Step 4: make a clinical decision
The assessment findings should give you enough information to identify pain prevention strategies that can be incorporated into Ken's care plan. This should include choice of a suitable dressing for Ken's wound that will enable him to have pain-free dressing changes and improved mobility.

Step 5: evaluate progress
Think about how you will reassess Ken's pain, comfort and mobility.

Suggested management

In the assessment of Ken's pain, he should be asked where the pain is, what it feels like, how long it has been like that and whether anything helps relieve or aggravates the pain. He should be asked to describe the pain in his own words and a suitable pain scale used to assess severity. Ken is anticipating that the dressing change will be painful and consequently he is anxious and frightened. Reassurance and building up a good rapport with patients is essential. Ken needs to feel confident that his concerns about the dressing change are being addressed. He should be given reassurance that the dressing procedure will be undertaken after he has had his analgesia and a different dressing will be applied that will not stick to his wound. It is important to check which analgesia he is taking and when it is next due. It is essential that Ken be given his prescribed analgesia prior to the dressing change, with a sufficient time gap for it to become effective.

The dressing choice should reflect the assessment findings. Ken has been experiencing pain at dressing changes and using appropriate dressings has been shown to be effective in the management of wound pain. A dressing such as soft silicone would be suitable as this does not adhere to the wound bed or surrounding skin and would allow Ken to have pain-free dressing changes. Ken should be reassured that the dressing will not cause him any discomfort from sticking or pulling on the wound. Retaining dressings in the groin area can be difficult and one solution would be the use of a pad and retention net pants. Ken could be given some pads to change himself as they become soiled and still leave his dressings in place. The treatment goal is to reduce Ken's pain at dressing changes and to improve his overall comfort and mobility. To evaluate the effectiveness of his treatment Ken's pain should be continually reassessed and changes in his pain scores documented. He should be asked if he is happy with the new dressing and whether he feels more comfortable. The dressing should continue to be comfortable for him and his mobility should continue to improve.

CONCLUSION

This exercise has shown you how to use a systematic approach in the assessment and management of a patient with wound pain.

REFERENCES

Briggs, M. (2006) The prevalence of pain in chronic wounds and nurses' awareness of the problem. *British Journal of Community Nursing* **15**(suppl)(21): 3–9.

Dunn, V. (2000) The holistic assessment of the patient in pain. *Professional Nurse* **15**: 791–793.

European Wound Management Association (2002) Position document. *Pain at Dressing Changes.* London, MEP Ltd.

Hofman, D. (2006a) Practical steps to address pain in wound care. Acknowledging and addressing chronic wound pain. *British Journal of Nursing* **15**(suppl)(21): 10–14.

Hofman, D. (2006b) Wound pain and dressings. In: White, R. & Harding, K. (eds) *Trauma and Pain in Wound Care.* Aberdeen, Wounds UK Ltd., p. 82.

Hollinworth, H. (2005) Pain at wound dressing-related procedures: a template for assessment. Available at: www.worldwidewounds.com/2005/august/Hollinworth/Framework-Assessing-Pain-Wound-Dressing-Related.html (accessed 3 Apr 2006).

Illich, I. (1976) *Medical Nemesis: the Exploration of Health.* Harmondsworth, Penguin Books.

Johnson, M. (2006) Physiology of pain. In: White, R. & Harding, K. (eds) *Trauma and Pain in Wound Care.* Aberdeen, Wounds UK Ltd., pp. 17–56.

Kiecolt-Glaser, J.K., Marucha, P.T., Malarkey, W.B., Mercado, A.M. & Glaser, R. (1995) Slowing of wound healing by psychological stress. *Larcet* **346**(8984): 1194–1196.

McCaffery, M. (1983) *Nursing the Patient in Pain.* London, Harper & Row.

McCaffery, M. & Pasero, C. (1999) *Pain: Clinical Manual.* St Louis, MO, Mosby.

McCaffery, M., Ferrell, B.R. & Pasero, C. (2000) Nurses personal opinions about patients' pain and their effect on recorded assessments and titration of opioid doses. *Pain Management Nursing* **1**(3): 79–87.

McGuire, L., Heffner, K., Glaser, R. *et al.* (2006) Pain and wound healing in surgical patients. *Annals of Behaviour Medicine* **31**(92): 165–172.

Melzack, R. & Wall, P.D. (1965) Pain mechanisms: a new theory. *Science* **150**: 971–979.

Melzack, R. & Wall, P.D. (1988) *The Challenge of Pain, Second Edition.* London, Penguin Books.

Merskey, H. & Bogduk, N. (1994) *Classification of Chronic Pain: Descriptions of Chronic Pain Syndromes and Definitions of Pain Terms, Second Edition.* Seattle, IASP Press.

Moffatt, C.J., Franks, P.J. & Hollinworth, H. (2002) Understanding wound pain and trauma: an international perspective. In: European Wound Management Association Position Document. *Pain at Dressing Changes.* London, Medical Education Partnership, pp. 2–7.

Ready, L. & Edwards, W.T. (1992) Management of acute pain: a practical guide. Seattle, IASP Press.

Turk, D.C. & Melzack, R. (2001) Preface. In: Turk, D. & Melzack, R. (eds) *Handbook of Pain Assessment.* New York, The Guildford Press.

World Union of Wound Healing Societies (2004) *Principles of Best Practice: Minimising Pain at Wound Dressing-Related Procedures.* London, MEP Ltd.

Quality of Life

INTRODUCTION

This chapter explores the different ways living with a chronic wound affects peoples' lives. Factors such as poor pain control, uncomfortable bandages and failure to manage exudate and odour can have a profound impact on a patient's quality of life. This chapter reviews some relevant literature in order to highlight problems reported by participants in quality-of-life (QoL) studies. The importance of listening to and working together with the patient to develop a plan of care that will reduce disruption to their life, increase their understanding of their condition and give them some element of control again is discussed.

HOW QUALITY OF LIFE IS MEASURED

Studies measuring QoL in a patient with a chronic wound have mainly focused on leg ulceration with a few studies looking at pressure ulcers using various methods of assessment. Generic measures of QoL can be used to examine how living with a chronic leg ulcer impacts on everyday living, within a set group of patients, compared with those in a population of similar age without leg ulcers (Price, 2001). Examples of recognised generic tools to measure QoL include the Symptom Rating Test (Franks *et al.*, 1994), the Nottingham Heath Profile and the Short Form 36 questionnaire (SF-36) (Lindholm *et al.*, 1993; Roe *et al.*, 1995;

Price & Harding, 1996; Franks & Moffatt, 2001). Other methods have included standardised personal interviews (Phillips *et al.*, 1994), condition-specific questionnaires (Price & Harding, 2004) and semi-structured interviews (Douglas, 2001; Rich & McLachlan, 2003). Some of these researchers have used several different methods.

PHYSICAL EXPERIENCES AND THEIR IMPACT ON DAILY LIVING

Both pressure ulcers and leg ulcers have been shown to have a significant impact on patients' QoL, with pain being an overwhelming feature. The pain experienced is not always attributed to the ulcer itself, however, with the topical treatment or the pressure redistributing mattress sometimes cited as the cause of the pain (Douglas, 2001; Briggs & Closs, 2006; Hopkins *et al.*, 2006; Spilsbury *et al.*, 2007). This can result in removal of the offending bandage or dressing after the nurse has left, when the patient has found the treatment to be too painful to continue with it. Patients may then become labelled as difficult or non-compliant. In a review on leg ulcers and their impact on daily life, Persoon *et al.* (2004) suggest that there is under-treatment of pain in patients with venous leg ulcers. Similar results have been found with patients with pressure ulcers (Spilsbury *et al.*, 2007). Pain associated with wounds is discussed in detail in Chapter 8.

Sleeplessness appears to be a major factor impacting on QoL and this is mainly associated with pain in the ulcer and general discomfort (Phillips *et al.*, 1994; Charles, 1995; Hareendran *et al.*, 2005; Spilsbury *et al.*, 2007). Bandages are often reported as being uncomfortable with some patients finding itching beneath the bandages a problem, which can lead to sleeplessness and irritability. Patients find mobility a problem and this is often influenced by pain, odour and leakage (Hareendran *et al.*, 2005). Restricted mobility has been reported as the reason for reduced social contact and difficulty in performing everyday tasks (Roe *et al.*, 1995). Patients find continuing to work a problem especially if it involves standing for long periods, which goes against the advice they have been given to rest their leg (Hyland *et al.*, 1994).

BODY IMAGE

Bathing and showering is difficult for patients with a leg ulcer, as they have to keep their bandages dry (Roe *et al.*, 1995; Douglas, 2001). This can leave them feeling dirty and reluctant to mix in company, which in turn increases their feelings of isolation. Wound leakage and odour present many problems. Concerns about wound exudate leaking into shoes and on to furniture and bedclothes are frequently expressed, resulting in anxiety and embarrassment (Phillips *et al.*, 1994; Walshe, 1995; Hyde *et al.*, 1999). Patients who are still working find trying to cope with leakage and odour particularly 'horrifying and distressing' (Douglas, 2001). Patients with a leg ulcer find their choice of clothes and footwear is often limited due to leakage or bulky compression bandages and female patients can feel self-conscious and have to resort to wearing trousers or long skirts to hide their legs. Embarrassment at having a leg ulcer can also have a damaging effect on intimacy (Rich & McLachlan, 2003; Hareendran *et al.*, 2005).

EMOTIONAL ASPECTS AND PERCEPTIONS

Many patients find that their life changes because of their ulcer and they are unable to undertake their usual role in the household or perform their usual tasks. Having to rely on other people to undertake the housework, do the garden or get the shopping leads to feelings of frustration and loss of identity. This can lead to loss of self-confidence, depression and a sense of hopelessness (Roe *et al.*, 1995; Douglas, 2001; Hareendran *et al.*, 2005; Hopkins *et al.*, 2006). Chronic wounds do not heal quickly and slow healing or lack of healing can be a source of frustration and depression for the patient. Patients are often concerned about whether they will have their ulcer for years, especially when another family member, maybe their mother, has been troubled by leg ulcers all their life. Some patients become resigned to having an ulcer and just get on with their life, with a sense of acceptance (Roe *et al.*, 1995; Douglas, 2001; Rich & McLachlan, 2003; Hopkins *et al.*, 2006). In a comparison of QoL in patients with acute or chronic wounds, there was a trend for patients with chronic wounds to rate their overall QoL higher than those with acute wounds. The authors suggest that this may be because patients with chronic wounds adapt to their condition over time (Price & Harding, 2000).

SOCIAL ASPECTS

There are various reasons why patients become isolated when they have a chronic leg ulcer. Reluctance to socialise due to leakage and odour from the wound has already been discussed. Another concern is worry about getting their legs knocked. The leg ulcer may have been caused by a knock in the first instance and the patient may be frightened of further injury or if the ulcer is healed they may be concerned that it may break down again if knocked. So they may be reluctant to go out or if there are small children in their family they may feel nervous about having them around as the children might knock against their leg.

TREATMENT PERCEPTIONS

Patients' perception of treatment is generally good but several studies have identified some areas of concern. The main issues patients have raised regarding their treatment are lack of continuity of care, nurses constantly changing the treatment and inconsistent advice. Lack of communication between patients and nurses has also been identified, with patients and carers having no understanding of the cause of their ulcer and little if any involvement in their treatment. There are frequent comments from patients on how busy the nurses are and that they have little time to talk – how they just rush in, do the dressing and leave. Patients have reported they are sometimes unable to comply with advice given because of other factors in their life. For example they may be given advice to rest with their leg elevated, but they may be the main carer for someone else and therefore cannot do so, or be the breadwinner and have to continue working in a job that involves a lot of standing (Hyland *et al.*, 1994; Walshe, 1995; Douglas, 2001; Rich & McLachlan, 2003).

PLANNING PATIENT CARE

Care should be holistic, focusing on the patient as well as the wound. Nursing practice in the management of chronic wounds should include wound care and appropriate adjunctive therapy together with consideration of patients' problems that affect their QoL. Good wound management practices that consider both the patient and the wound have been shown to significantly improve patients QoL (Charles, 2004).

It is important that nurses listen to their patients and address their concerns when working with them to develop a plan of care. Douglas (2001) suggests that a collaborative approach between the patient and nurse leads to more control in a patient's life and improved self-esteem. Patients would like to be more involved in their care and to be able to make choices about their treatment. To be able to do this they need to be well informed. Patient information leaflets are a valuable resource and relevant material should be readily available to all patients. It is important that as a nurse you develop good communication skills and ensure that you have a good working knowledge of how different dressings perform, and the benefits of any appropriate adjunctive therapy, e.g. compression therapy, to enable you to discuss patients' care with them. The terminology you use should be expressed in a form that the patient is able to understand. When you are working together with the patient to develop a plan of care you will also need to consider the ability of the patient to communicate, product availability in your area of work and any cost implications (Vowden & Vowden, 2006). Patients have raised concerns about nurses constantly changing their treatment and of being given conflicting advice. If patients have a bad treatment experience this can result in them losing confidence and belief in their treatment. Patients need to have confidence in the nurses who are treating them and the treatment being administered. To maintain continuity and consistency of care it is essential that all clinical decision-making and advice given to the patient are evidence based and clinical guidelines are adhered to. Any changes to their treatment should first be discussed with the patient and a reason given to them for the change. Clear documentation identifying the rationale for the change can help avoid unnecessary changes in future. When evaluating how the wound is healing you should also evaluate any adjunctive therapy and the feelings and experiences of the patient. Thus you will ensure that the treatment you have instigated is comfortable and acceptable to the patient enabling them to continue with their life with as little disruption as possible.

Key points
- Wounds such as leg ulcers have been shown to have a significant impact on patients' QoL.
- Pain in the ulcer is the most overwhelming feature.
- Sleeplessness, poor mobility, embarrassment, isolation and difficulty with personal hygiene have all been reported to adversely affect patients' QoL.
- Patients are often unable to undertake their usual role in the household or perform their usual tasks, leaving them frustrated and anxious.
- Concerns about treatment include lack of continuity of care, nurses constantly changing treatments and inconsistent or unrealistic advice.
- All care should be holistic, focusing on the patient as well as the wound.

Continued

- Ensure patients have adequate information about their condition.
- Listen to the patient and address their concerns.
- Develop a plan of care with the patient.
- Regularly evaluate the wound, the suitability of the compression levels and the feelings and experiences of the patient.

SUMMARY

This chapter has identified how living with a chronic wound such as a leg ulcer can negatively affect a person's quality of life. By adopting a collaborative approach with their patients when developing their plan of care, nurses can go a long way in improving their patients' QoL. Identifying and addressing problems related to QoL should be incorporated in the care plan.

You should now use the knowledge you have gained from reading this chapter to undertake the following exercise.

Exercise 9.1

Case scenario

Mrs White is a 78-year-old lady with a long history of venous leg ulcers. She was successfully healed 2 years ago, but 4 months ago one ulcer re-occurred. Mrs White has been reassessed and her ABPI found to be 0.95. Her ulcer was responding to treatment with a non-adherent dressing and layered compression bandaging,

Continued

changed weekly. Mrs White is aware that recently the ulcer has become malodorous and now her bandages are stained. She says that her family normally visit twice a week, but her daughter came alone yesterday. Her granddaughters did not visit her, as they 'do not like the smell of granny's leg'. She is very upset about this and feels isolated.

Using a systematic approach, think about what may be causing the malodour and how this may be resolved to improve Mrs White's quality of life.

Step 1: assess the patient, wound and circumstances
Consider any changes that may have occurred to cause the malodour.
What will you ask Mrs White?

Step 2: utilise existing information about the patient
Consider the underlying aetiology of her ulcer.

Step 3: explore relevant current best practice
Consider how important compression bandaging is, how appropriate the dressing is and expectations of wear time.

Step 4: make a clinical decision
You should now have enough information to determine what may be causing the malodour and to write a treatment plan that includes the impact on Mrs White's QoL.

Step 5: evaluate progress
How would you continue to evaluate Mrs White's QoL.

Suggested management

Mrs White's ulcer was healing but her quality of life then deteriorated due to malodour of her ulcer. You should ask Mrs White how long it was after the ulcer was dressed before there was any odour. Bandage staining suggests an increase in exudate production. Mrs White should be asked about her pain levels, as increased exudate and increased wound pain are an indication of infection requiring medical advice.

It may be that she is more active than usual or that the dressing is left too long between changes. The wound should be reassessed and a dressing that provides an optimum moisture balance selected. The frequency of dressing changes may influence the level of malodour and thus may need to be carefully monitored for a while.

Her treatment should adhere to relevant clinical guidelines and the most important factor in the management of venous leg ulcers is compression. This should be continued and periods of leg elevation encouraged. Ongoing evaluation of the patient and the wound ensures that appropriate changes are made in light of changing circumstances, thus improving the patient's QoL.

CONCLUSION

This exercise has shown you how to work through the decision-making process in a systematic way.

REFERENCES

Briggs, M. & Closs, S.J. (2006) Patients perceptions of the impact of treatments and products on their experience of leg ulcer pain. *Journal of Wound Care* **15**: 333–337.

Charles, H. (1995) The impact of leg ulcers on patients' quality of life. *Professional Nurse* **10**: 571–573.

Charles, H. (2004) Does leg ulcer treatment improve patients' quality of life? *Journal of Wound Care* **13**: 209–215.

Douglas, V. (2001) Living with a chronic leg ulcer: an insight into patients' experiences and feelings. *Journal of Wound Care* **10**: 355–360.

Franks, P.J. & Moffatt, C.J. (2001) Health related quality of life in patients with venous ulceration: use of the Nottingham Health Profile. *Quality of Life Research* **10**: 693–700.

Franks, P.J., Moffatt, C.J., Connolly, M., Bosanquet, N., Oldryd, M., Greenhalgh, R.M. & McCollum, C.N. (1994) Community leg ulcer clinics: effect on quality of life. *Phlebology* **9**: 83–86.

Hareendran, A., Bradbury, A., Budd, J., Geroulakos, G., Hobbs, R., Kenkre, J. & Symonds, T. (2005) Measuring the impact of venous ulcers on quality of life. *Journal of Wound Care* **14**: 53–57.

Hopkins, A., Dealey, C., Bale, S., Defloor, T. & Worboys, F. (2006) Patient stories of living with a pressure ulcer. *Journal of Advanced Nursing* **56**(4): 345–353.

Hyde, C., Ward, B., Horsfall, J. & Winder, G. (1999) Older women's experience of living with chronic leg ulceration. *International Journal of Nursing Practice* **5**: 189–198.

Hyland, M.E., Ley, A. & Thompson, B. (1994) Quality of life of leg ulcer patients: questionnaire and preliminary findings. *Journal of Wound Care* **3**: 294–298.

Lindholm, C., Bjellerup, M., Christensen, O.B. & Zederfeldt, B. (1993) Quality of life in chronic leg ulcer patients. *Acta Dermato-venereologica* **73**: 440–443.

Persoon, A., Heinen, M.M., van der Vleuten, C.J.M., de Rooij, M.J., van der Kerkhof, P.C.M. & van Achterberg, T. (2004) Leg ulcers: a review of their impact on daily life. *Journal of Clinical Nursing* **13**: 341–354.

Phillips, T., Stanton, B., Provan, A. & Lew, R. (1994) A study of the impact of leg ulcers on quality of life: financial, social and psychologic implications. *Journal of the American Academy of Dermatology* **31**: 49–53.

Price, P. (2001) Quality of life. In: Krasner, D.L., Rodeheaver, G.T. & Sibbald, R.G. (eds) *Chronic Wound Care: A Clinical Source Book for Healthcare Professionals, Third Edition.* Wayne, PA, HMP Communications.

Price, P. & Harding, K. (1996) Measuring health-related quality of life in patients with chronic leg ulcers. *Wounds* **8**: 91–94.

Price, P. & Harding, K.G. (2000) Acute and chronic wounds: differences in self-reported health-related quality of life. *Journal of Wound Care* **9**: 93–95.

Price, P. & Harding, K. (2004) Cardiff wound impact schedule: the development of a condition-specific questionnaire to assess health-related quality of life in patients with chronic wounds of the lower limb. *International Wound Journal* **1**: 10–17.

Rich, A. & McLachlan, L. (2003) How living with a leg ulcer affects people's daily life: a nurse-led study. *Journal of Wound Care* **12**: 51–55.

Roe, B., Cullum, N. & Hunter, C. (1995) Patients' perceptions of chronic leg ulceration. In: Cullum, N. & Roe, B. (eds) *Leg Ulcers: Nursing Management. A Research Based Guide.* Middlesex, Scutari Press.

Spilsbury, K., Nelson, A., Cullum, N., Iglesias, C., Nixon, J. & Mason, S. (2007) Pressure ulcers and their treatment and effects on quality of life: hospital inpatient perspectives. *Journal of Advanced Nursing* **57**(5): 494–504.

Vowden, K. & Vowden, P. (2006) Bridging the gap: the impact of patient choice on wound care. *Journal of Wound Care* **15**: 143–145.

Walshe, C. (1995) Living with a venous ulcer: a descriptive study of patients' experiences. *Journal of Advanced Nursing* **22**: 1092–1100.

Using a Systematic Approach to Managing a Complex Wound

INTRODUCTION

The purpose of this book is to provide basic information on the management of all types of commonly found wounds. In this concluding chapter, the aim is to bring together all the knowledge you have gained from reading this book. Throughout the book there are case scenarios that gradually built on what you have learnt in each chapter, where you have been guided to use a systematic approach to help you determine your response. That same format is used in this chapter to address the management of a complex wound.

WHAT IS A COMPLEX WOUND?

A complex wound is one that does not heal in a straightforward way, but is prone to complication or requires multiple interventions and takes a long time to heal. It is likely that a number of different healthcare professionals will be involved in the management of a complex wound.

The following exemplar will demonstrate how to manage a patient with a complex wound.

EXEMPLAR
Patient history
Mrs Bolton is a 59-year-old woman with multiple sclerosis (MS), who cannot move her legs and has little sense of feeling in them. She is able to move her arms but her movements tend to be jerky and are not well controlled. She has gradually become more dependent and spends most days just sitting in her wheelchair reading and watching television. Her husband is 10 years older than she is and is her main carer. Mr Bolton still manages to take his wife out for walks in her wheelchair when the weather is warm enough. He also does all the shopping, cooking and household chores. They have one daughter who lives abroad. Mr and Mrs Bolton have been self-sufficient for many years, but recently Mr Bolton has not been coping very well with looking after his wife. In order to provide him with some support, Mrs Bolton has been offered a place in a nurse-led hospital-based day centre, which she can attend either 2 or 3 days per week, and both she and her husband are considering accepting this. Mrs Bolton's appetite has become generally poor, mainly because it takes her so long to eat a meal. She has recently lost some weight. Over the past few months Mrs Bolton has started to slump slightly to one side and her right leg has been pressing against the leg of the wheelchair, causing pressure on her calf. She still sleeps well at night and her usual sleeping position is on her back. She has developed a wound on the back of her right calf that has been present for several weeks.

The wound

The wound is necrotic in the centre with some granulation tissue present at the edges (Fig. 10.1). The wound has slowly increased in diameter, but it is difficult to determine the depth of this wound due to the amount of necrotic tissue present. The wound is exuding and there is also a noticeable malodour that is distressing for both the patient and her husband.

A systematic approach is now used to help you in the process of assessing this patient and her wound and in planning the most appropriate care.

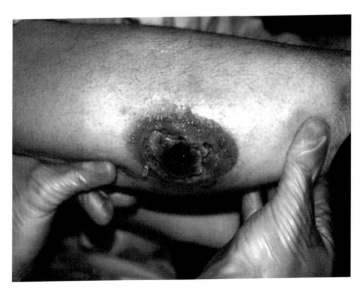

Fig. 10.1 Ulcer at initial assessment.

Step 1: assess the patient, wound and circumstances

Your assessment of the patient should include the general health of the patient, any concomitant medical conditions, medication, risk factors and social factors. Mrs Bolton has MS and because of her immobility and because she has little feeling in her legs she is at risk from injury to them. In addition her arm movements are jerky and not well controlled and she is at risk of dropping things onto her legs.

Your assessment of the wound should include the following:

• What factors were involved in the development of this wound?

It is often useful to determine the aetiology of the wound as in this case. The wound is a pressure ulcer caused by poor positioning resulting in Mrs Bolton's right calf pressing against her wheelchair.

• Where is the wound on the body?

It is important to record the exact position of a wound as the patient may have other wounds with different aetiologies. The position of the wound may also affect dressing choice and positioning of the patient. This wound is a pressure ulcer on the back of her right leg on the calf. Therefore an essential component of management of this wound is to remove the pressure source.

• How long has it been there?

The patient or relatives may be able to tell you when they first noticed the wound and how it has changed.

- What does it look like?

Many clinical areas have developed their own specific charts for wound assessment. Good documentation is essential in order for all members of the team caring for the patient to obtain a clear picture of the wound. This will form the basis for future assessments and evaluation of progress.

On examination, there is a black/brown 'plug' of necrotic tissue in the centre with a small rim of granulation tissue at the wound edges. The colour and viscosity of the exudate should be carefully noted, as increased levels of exudate and discoloration might indicate the presence of infection. Normal wound exudate is a pale straw colour in appearance. The peri-ulcer skin is intact and needs protecting as the wound is exuding and the skin may become macerated.

The wound should be measured, and this information dated and incorporated into the wound assessment documentation so that it can be used to compare against later measurements.

Step 2: utilise existing information about the patient
Using information you already have about the patient you should consider the following.

- Is this wound affecting the patient's quality of life?

The main concern for the patient is the malodour and this can be addressed by assessment of the wound and the appropriate dressing.

- Has anything changed recently?

It is important that holistic assessment of the patient with a wound should include nutritional screening as nutrient deficiencies can adversely affect healing. Mrs Bolton's appetite has decreased and consequently she has lost weight. In addition, her positioning in her wheelchair has changed because she has difficulty in sitting up straight, and this must be addressed.

- Who are the carers?

Are the patient's carers able to cope or do they require additional help? Mrs Bolton is becoming more dependent on her husband and as he is getting older he is finding it more difficult to cope. Mr and Mrs Bolton should be given as much information as possible about the day centre and the benefits of the care she will receive there to help her and her husband make an informed decision about accepting the place they have been offered.

- Is the patient in an appropriate wheelchair?

When was the last time Mrs Bolton had an assessment of the appropriateness of her wheelchair? The day care centre would be able to undertake an assessment of Mrs Bolton's needs and make an appropriate referral.

Does she require support in the chair to help her to sit in a better position? Again, this could be assessed at the day centre.

Step 3: explore relevant current best practice
Explore current recommendations and guidelines for wound debridement. 'You should always base your treatment decisions on good evidence'. Check if there are any local guidelines for wound debridement within your working area. The NICE pressure ulcer treatment guidelines (NICE, 2005) provide advice on

the debridement of pressure ulcers, so are a good start-ing point.

Step 4: make a clinical decision

Once a full assessment of both the patient and the wound have been completed, it is possible to plan the most appropriate care. This should include how you will debride this wound. You should also include how you expect the wound will look after it has been debrided, the type of dressing that will be required and any skin care regimen.

• Wound and skin care

You should set short-term achievable goals. A suitable debridement method such as larval therapy should be applied to remove the necrotic material and reduce odour. The wound will become very different after larval therapy. The wound shape and depth will change as necrotic material is removed and replaced by granulation tissue. Once the necrotic tissue starts to break down, exudate levels may increase requir-ing more frequent dressing changes. A suitable skin protectant such as zinc oxide paste or a protective skin wipe should be applied around the wound to protect the peri-ulcer skin from damage from exudate. Your immediate goals in managing this wound are, there-fore, to remove the necrotic material so that healthy granulation tissue can form and to maintain peri-ulcer skin integrity.

• Who else may be involved in the care of the patient?

As Mrs Bolton has a poor dietary intake she would benefit from advice from a dietician. She should also have an appropriate referral for assessment of her wheelchair requirements and other pressure aids such as a cushion. Referral routes may vary according to local healthcare provision.

Step 5: evaluate progress
Ongoing reassessment of the wound and evaluation of the treatment will ensure that timely changes are made to optimise a successful outcome.

Following initial debridement the wound should be reassessed, as it may well become an exuding cavity wound (see Fig. 10.2). An appropriate dressing at this

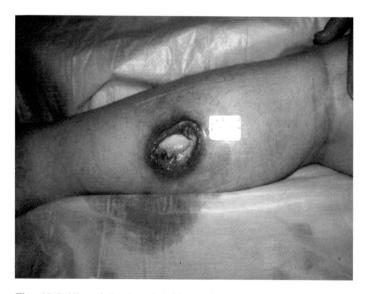

Fig. 10.2 Ulcer following debridement.

stage would be an alginate rope or hydrofibre packing as either of these would fill the cavity and absorb the exudate. Assessment of the amount of wound exudate may be determined by assessing the interaction with the dressing. Any changes in levels or appearance should be recorded as this may influence the continued suitability of the dressing or frequency of dressing changes.

CONCLUSION

The aim of this book has been to provide the reader with information about basic aspects of wound management. However, this is only the start of the journey. True expertise in wound management can only be attained by applying this theory to practice, acquiring further knowledge of specific wounds and by observing and managing a wide range of wounds. This will take time and it is important to recognise that the journey is never complete as there is always more to learn. But there can be great rewards along the way.

REFERENCES

National Institute for Health and Clinical Excellence and Royal College of Nursing (2005) *The Management of Pressure Ulcers in Primary and Secondary Care*. London, NICE.

Index

Note: page numbers in *italics* refer to figures and boxes, those in **bold** refer to tables